OTOLARYNGOLOGY RESEARCH ADVANCES

PARATHYROID

ANATOMY, FUNCTIONS AND DISORDERS

Otolaryngology Research Advances

Additional books in this series can be found on Nova's website under the Series tab.

Additional e-books in this series can be found on Nova's website under the e-book tab.

Human Anatomy and Physiology

Additional books in this series can be found on Nova's website under the Series tab.

Additional e-books in this series can be found on Nova's website under the e-book tab.

OTOLARYNGOLOGY RESEARCH ADVANCES

PARATHYROID

ANATOMY, FUNCTIONS AND DISORDERS

JAMES KIRKBY-BOTT

EDITOR

Nova Science Publishers, Inc.

New York

For permission to use material from this book please contact us:
Telephone 631-231-7269; Fax 631-231-8175
Web Site: http://www.novapublishers.com

NOTICE TO THE READER

Additional color graphics may be available in the e-book version of this book.

Library of Congress Cataloging-in-Publication Data

Parathyroid : anatomy, functions, and disorders / editor, James Kirkby-Bott.
p. ; cm.
Includes bibliographical references and index.
ISBN 978-1-62100-765-4 (hardcover)
I. Kirkby-Bott, James.
[DNLM: 1. Parathyroid Diseases. 2. Parathyroid Glands. WK 300]
616.4'45--dc23

2011038562

Published by Nova Science Publishers, Inc. † New York

Contents

Preface

This book follows an up to date authoritative style on the subject of parathyroid glands and their disorder. This book seeks to expand the horizon of parathyroid hormone use and provides in depth information on surgical techniques for managing its disorder. There are four sections on anatomy, function, disorder and treatment. The first three show how these areas are interconnected and the fourth on techniques for managing parathyroid disease. While short enough to be read as a treatise on parathyroid glands it is also authorative enough to be used as a reference text.

Chapter 1 - A thorough knowledge of the embryology and anatomy of the parathyroid glands is mandatory for every surgeon aiming to perform thyroid and parathyroid surgery with low morbidity and high chances of success. The superior and inferior parathyroid glands derive from the fourth and third branchial pouches, respectively.

The superior glands have a short migratory path and final location near the middle thyroid lobe. The inferior parathyroid glands are located at the lower thyroid lobe in more than 50% but their long migratory pathway predisposes them to frequent ectopic positions, especially in the upper thymus. The arterial supply of the parathyroid glands is terminal in type. The vascularization of inferior parathyroid glands depends primarily on the inferior thyroid artery. The inferior thyroid artery also supplies the superior parathyroid glands in 80-90%. 15% are supplied by a posterior branch of the superior thyroid artery, or by the posterior marginal arch of Evans. Parathyroid gland venous drainage reaches one of the three thyroid veins via the venous complex along the thyroid capsule and its damage leads to transient hypoparathyroidism.

Chapter 2 - The purpose of imaging of the parathyroid glands is mainly for localisation of the abnormal gland(s) and pre-operative surgical planning. A number of imaging modalities are available, each with its own indications, advantages and disadvantages. However, given that surgical intervention is still the treatment of most parathyroid diseases and that minimally invasive surgery in localised primary hyperparathyroidism is becoming the gold standard, the importance of imaging takes on a paramount value: to avoid unsuccessful explorative surgery.

Normal parathyroid glands are not normally seen on most imaging modalities, given that their mean size is 6x4x2mm[1,2]. However, in the diseased state, be that an adenoma, carcinoma or hyperplasia, the glands become distinct from their surrounding structures, and can be identified more readily. Further, of the four parathyroid glands - two superior and particularly the two inferior, ectopic locations are not uncommon. As part of pre-operative planning it is essential that ectopic glands are identified, and the newer imaging modalities can identify such glands quite accurately. The ectopic location may be as diverse as the retro-oesophageal space, the mediastinum, or even the skull base as described in chapter 1. Also, 5% of patients may have supernumerary glands, and both clinician and radiologist should be alert to this [3,4]. Importantly, it is useful to remember that imaging forms only a part of the investigative and management process that is essential to treat parathyroid disease. Clinical and family history, biochemical studies and imaging all contribute to the development of a diagnosis, which allows the endocrinologist or surgeon to ably treat these diseases. Whilst ultrasound and sestamibi are routinely used in localisation other modalities are increasing interest, particularly when ultrasound and sestamibi have been unable to localise the diseased gland. The purpose of this chapter is to describe the main imaging techniques available for the assessment of diseased parathyroid glands, or as part of investigation into deranged biochemical function. The uses, indications, advantages and pitfalls of each modality are discussed.

Chapter 3 - The parathyroid glands located in the neck, secrete parathyroid hormone (PTH) which is a key player in calcium homeostasis and bone health. The regulation of calcium homeostasis involves the interactions of PTH, Vitamin-D, calcitonin, and serum calcium with the latter acting via the calcium sensing receptor (CaSR).

In this chapter the histology of the parathyroid glands, structure of PTH, challenges in biochemical measurement of PTH, the structure and role of the calcium sensing receptor (CaSR), and the functional mutations in the CaSR contributing to disease models are explored. The role of Calcitonin in calcium metabolism and regulation of PTH secretion and action is reviewed.

Parathyroid related protein structure, secretion and its place in the diagnostic pathway for hypercalcaemia are discussed. Finally the mechanisms underlying hypocalcaemia and hypoparathyroidism and the clinical picture, management and monitoring is outlined.

Chapter 4 – Parathyroid hormone (PTH) plays a central role in the regulation of calcium and phosphate homeostasis. PTH acts directly increasing renal calcium reabsorption and phosphate excretion and indirectly enhancing intestinal calcium absorption. Continuous exposure to exogenous PTH causes an increase in bone resorption, whereas, bone formation is stimulated when PTH is delivered intermittently. There are two areas of research with intermittent PTH application - improvement of bone tissue and the use of PTH to enhance bone repair after fracture. Currently, human parathyroid hormone (hPTH 1-84) and its analog, recombinant hPTH 1-34, are being used for treatment of severe osteoporosis in humans. However, this treatment has significant limitations related to its daily subcutaneous administration and high costs. Little data exist on the effect of PTH treatments of different durations and regimes. The chapter is focused on the effect of PTH on bone tissue either intact or injured in healthy or osteoporotic subjects applied at different regimes and durations.

Evaluation of the lumbar vertebral region is also extremely important because of its high clinical relevance in the treatment of osteoporosis. In a series of experiments, three-month old rats developed osteoporotic changes after ovariectomy during 8 weeks, healthy rats were left intact. Thereafter, all rats underwent bilateral transverse osteotomy in tibia metaphysis (day 0) and were treated with PTH applied at different regimes.

After 35 post-osteotomy days their lumbar spine was analyzed. The first lumbar vertebral body (L1) was used for histological analysis, L2 for computed tomographic (CT) analysis, L3 was ashed and L4 was used for biomechanical testing. In the first trial, five-week daily PTH treatment improved cortical and cancellous bone parameters in lumbar spine in ovariectomy induced osteopenic rats (Ovx).

Chapter 5 – Primary hyperparathyroidism is a common endocrine condition and in 1:10 patients it can occur as part of the recognised familial endocrine cancer syndromes - rare inherited autosomal dominant diseases with high penetrance. Identification of patients with familial PHPT is important for two main reasons. Firstly, the affected patients may be at risk from tumours that may arise in different glands, and regular screening for these tumours together with earlier treatment is expected to improve their prognosis. Secondly, the relatives of an affected patient are at a 50% risk of having inherited the mutation and thus developing such tumours.

These syndromes include multiple endocrine neoplasia type 1 (MEN1) and type 2 (MEN2), familial isolated primary hyperparathyroidism (FIHP), the hyperpara-thyroidism-jaw tumour syndrome (HPT-JT), familial benign hypocalciuric hypercalcaemia (FHH) and neonatal primary hyperparathyroidism (NHPT). Compared with sporadic PHPR, familial cases present at a younger age, are associated with multiglandular involvement and have a higher tendency to recur. The clinical features and their diagnosis, investigations and genetics, and management of each of these syndromes will be reviewed.

Chapter 6 - Childhood parathyroid disorders are rare phenomena. Primary, Secondary and Tertiary hyperparathyroidism can occur in children and adolescents in a similar manner as to in adults, though in primary HPT they are more likely to have a familial syndrome. Neonatal and childhood hypoparathyroid occurs due to: inherited genetic syndromes, gland damage during neck surgery, copper deposition or exposure to ionising radiation. Preterm infants are at risk of a transient hypoparathyroid hypocalcaemia. Children can present with acute symptoms such as tetany, cardiac conduction abnormalities and GI upset. Autoimmune causes can be associated with adrenal insufficiency which needs to be looked for in the assessment of these patients.

Chapter 7 – Parathyroid carcinoma (PC) accounts for less than 1% of cases of sporadic primary hyperparathyroidism (PHPT) and is usually associated with more severe clinical manifestations than parathyroid adenoma. Its course is typically indolent, but progressive. The diagnosis of malignancy is often made only when local recurrence or metastases occur, because the histology of parathyroid tumors can be equivocal or frankly misleading. Surgery is the only curative treatment for PC and consists of complete resection of the primary lesion at the time of initial operation. For this reason, both preoperative suspicion and intraoperative recognition are of great importance. Despite a potentially curative resection, PC has a recurrence rate of more than 50%. Most recurrences occur 2-3 years after the initial operation, but this period is variable and a prolonged disease-free interval of as long as 20 years has been reported. Most patients with recurrent disease ultimately succumb to the effects of hypercalcemia, rather than to direct tumor invasion or distant metastases. Recently, the calcimimetic cinacalcet, an allosteric modulator of the calcium sensing receptor, has be effectively employed to control hypercalcemia in patients with metastatic disease in whom surgical options were exhausted.

Chapter 8 - Primary hyperparathyroidism is an uncommon clinical entity with a variable worldwide incidence. The incidence and mode of presentation has changed with advances in biochemical assays. Most patients in the West now present earlier diagnosed on biochemical assay results rather than gross physical signs and radiology changes. Neuro-psychiatric symptoms with their insidious onset have become the most common presenting complaint.

The development of intact PTH assays and quick PTH assays as well as ultrasound, Sestamibi and most recently 4D triphasic CT scanning has altered the surgical approach and improved surgical outcomes so that 95% of patients are cured at surgery.

Chapter 9 – Advances in the accuracy of preoperative and peri-operative localizing techniques has lead to a preference for a minimally invasive procedure over bilateral exploration in image localized sporadic primary hyperparathyroidism. The focused approach has been shown to be equivalent to bilateral exploration for cure rate and superior to it concerning cosmetic result, duration of the intervention, postoperative stay, and hypocalcaemia, as assessed by prospective and randomized trials. [61, 62]. During the last decade, multiple minimally invasive approaches have been described [63], including: minimally invasive open parathyroidectomy, endoscopic and video-assisted parathyroidectomy and extra-cervical access from incisions in the chest wall and/or axilla.

The first endoscopic parathyroidectomy was described initially by Gagner in 1996. Minimally invasive video-assisted parathyroidectomy was first described by Miccoli et al. [47], and totally endoscopic parathyroidectomy by the lateral approach by Henry et al. [13]. Currently the best indication for the latter approach is adenomas that lie deep to the thyroid lobe, usually arising from superior gland adenomas.

All these minimally invasive techniques rely on preoperative localizing studies and may benefit from intra-operative PTH monitoring in certain scenarios as shown by Barczynski et al. [64]. The major problem with endoscopic parathyroidectomy is the limited working space so that associated nodular thyroid disease and the presence of a large (3 cm) parathyroid adenoma are relative contraindications. It has also been difficult to show a real advantage for endoscopic versus open minimally invasive surgery, largely due to the expense of the endoscopic equipment required. In 2006 Barczynski published a prospective, randomized trial on open versus video-assisted techniques [38]. This showed a preference in the minimally invasive video assisted parathyroidectomy (MIVAP) group due to an easier recognition of the recurrent laryngeal nerve, less postoperative pain and a better cosmetic results. On the other hand, there was a significantly higher operative cost. [65]

This chapter will shed the light on these different procedures along with the indications, limitations, and adavantages.

Chapter 10- Secondary and tertiary HPT are consequences of renal failure. 1,25 Vitamin D deficiency is associated with parathyroid hyperplasia and is a consequence of renal failure as conversion from 25 OH cholecalciferol to 1,25 dihydroxycholecalciferol, the active form of vitamin D, occurs in the renal parenchyma.

Secondary and Tertiary HPT refer to nodular multigland hyperplasia with excessive over secretion of PTH. This causes ectopic calcification and bone demineralization and hastens declining renal function due to nephrocalcinosis, causing concern for subsequent graft function in transplanted patients who have excessive PTH production at the time of surgery and or develop tertiary HPT post transplantation. Medical treatment with calcimimetics has not been as successful as first hoped and surgery remains the cornerstone treatment of secondary HPT.

There is debate as to the best surgical strategy sub-total parathyroidectomy and total parathyroidectomy +/- auto transplantation and cryopreservation of parathyroid tissue all have their own benefits and drawbacks.

Chapter 11- Re-operation for persistent or recurrent hyperparathyroidism can present significant challenges. Predictive factors of ectopic parathyroid gland location and failure of imaging in patients with persistent or recurrent hyperparathyroidism are reviewed. Ectopic gland location is frequent in re-operative disease with a reported incidence of 23-77%. Multivariate analysis identified secondary and persistent disease as predictors of ectopic glands (all ectopic locations).

Renal HPT patients were more prone to have ectopic glands while those with concomitant thyroid pathology less likely to have mediastinal glands. Secondary disease and high number of previously removed glands were associated with a thymic location. Ultrasound failure is higher in ectopic glands, secondary HPT predicts sestamibi failure and ectopic location was a predictor of combined ultrasound and sestamibi failure. Combined selective venous sampling and parathyroid angiography have an accuracy rate of 95%.

Meticulous pre-operative investigation is crucial for successful treatment of patients with persistent and recurrent hyperparathyroidism. The identified factors are useful for interpreting imaging results and planning surgical strategy in re-operations and they give insight into reasons for failure that help define a strategy when dealing with difficult initial operations. Such factors are very useful for interpreting imaging results and planning operative strategy in this group of patients.

Part 1:
Parathyroid Anatomy

In: Parathyroid: Anatomy, Functions and Disorders
Editor: James Kirkby-Bott
ISBN: 978-1-62100-765-4

Chapter I

Parathyroid Anatomy and Embryology

Bassam Abboud, Ronald Daher, and James Kirkby-Bott
[1]Department of General Surgery, Hotel-Dieu de Farnce Hospital,
Faculty of Medicine, Saint-Joseph University, Beirut-Lebanon
[2] Kingston Hospital, Surrey, UK

Abstract

A thorough knowledge of the embryology and anatomy of the parathyroid glands is mandatory for every surgeon aiming to perform thyroid and parathyroid surgery with low morbidity and high chances of success. The superior and inferior parathyroid glands derive from the fourth and third branchial pouches, respectively.

The superior glands have a short migratory path and final location near the middle thyroid lobe. The inferior parathyroid glands are located at the lower thyroid lobe in more than 50% but their long migratory pathway predisposes them to frequent ectopic positions, especially in the upper thymus. The arterial supply of the parathyroid glands is terminal in type. The vascularization of inferior parathyroid glands depends primarily on the inferior thyroid artery. The inferior thyroid artery also supplies the superior parathyroid glands in 80-90%. 15% are supplied by a posterior branch of the superior thyroid artery, or by the posterior marginal arch of Evans. Parathyroid gland venous drainage reaches one of the three thyroid veins via the venous complex along the thyroid capsule and its damage leads to transient hypoparathyroidism.

Introduction

Surgery for hyperparathyroidism should be ruled by two main principles: minimal morbidity and a 95% chance of restoring normocalcemia. Additionally, knowledge of parathyroid vascularisation makes thyroid surgery safer by reducing the risk of hypocalcaemia. This can only be achieved by thorough knowledge of the basic sciences such as embryology, anatomy and vascularization as they apply to the parathyroid glands.

Embryology

Parathyroid glands are endodermal in origin with tissue differentiation starting in the fifth developmental week, [1, 2, 3]. The superior parathyroid glands derive from the dorsal wing of the fourth branchial pouch.

During the seventh week of development this complex migrates towards the lateral border of the principal median thyroid diverticulum that derives from the ventral portion of the first and second pharyngeal pouches elongating along its caudal descent into the thyroglossal tract. This forms a bilobed structure anterior or ventral to the hyoid bone and laryngeal cartilages. These lobes become the left and right thyroid lobes joined by the thyroid isthmus. Consequently, the cervical migration path of the superior glands is relatively short and the superior parathyroid glands remain close to the supero-posterior aspect of the thyroid lobes [5].

The inferior parathyroid glands derive from the dorsal part of the third branchial pouch while the anterior part gives rise to the thymus [4]. They detach together from the pharyngeal wall and head in a caudal direction towards the superior mediastinum due to the cervical deflexion and migration of the heart and main vessels [6].

It is the thymic part that causes the large caudal migration of the inferior parathyroid glands. During the eighth week of development, the cephalad regression of the thymus leaves the inferior parathyroid glands at the lower part of the thyroid lobes or within the thyrothymic ligament.

As a result, the inferior parathyroid gland crosses the superior one during migration, and depending on its stopping point, the ipsilateral superior and inferior parathyroid glands can be close to each other or far apart. It is worth noting at this point the other derivatives of the third and fourth arches as this enlightens us as to the potential ectopic resting points of parathyroid glands.

The third arch derivatives include the greater and inferior parts of the hyoid bone and stylopharyngeus muscle. The fourth arch derivatives comprise the pharyngeal and laryngeal structures. Using this model to account for ectopy the fate of the branchial arch arteries also helps to account for some of anomalies described.

The third arch artery continues as part of the internal carotid artery so that the very rare cases of parathyroid glands being found in the carotid sheath are probably inferior parathyroid glands, whilst the fourth arch artery persists on the right as a part of the subclavian artery and on the left as arch of the aorta helping to explain how some superior glands can reach down to the aorto-pulmonary window. The path of the third branchial arch artery also extends down to the aortic arch so mediastinal glands could arise from the superior or inferior parathyroid (figure 1.1).

From this we can see how the variation in position of the parathyroid can range from the skull base near the pharyngeal wall origins and down to and beyond the aorto-pulmonary window in the thorax. In parathyroid hyperplasia ectopic parathyroid tissue can be found along the migratory pathway of the inferior parathyroid where a few cells have been stimulated to enlargement and proliferation. While there are no major series reporting on the effect of abnormal migration of related anatomy and parathyroid location it would be reasonable to assume there may be some influence on parathyroid position in such rare cases.

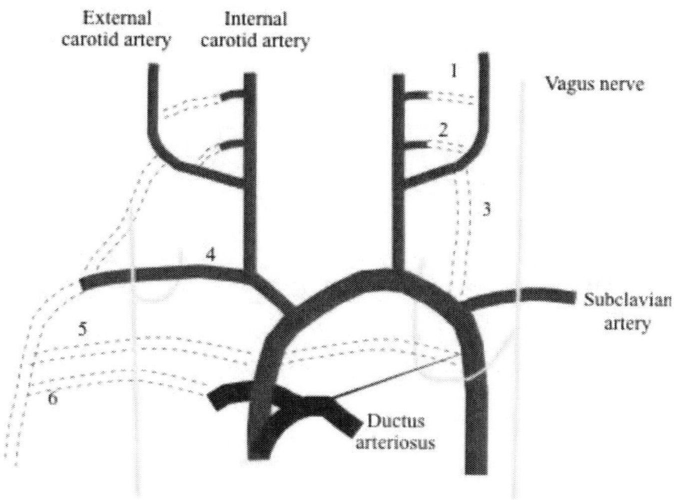

Figure 1.1. Branchial arch positions in the developing fetus superimposed on adult anatomical landmarks.

Topographic Anatomy

The relatively short migratory path of the superior parathyroid glands guarantees a more stable final location in comparison to the inferior parathyroid glands. In 85% of cases, they are found at the posterior aspect of thyroid lobes in a 1cm-radius circular area centered just above the intersection of inferior thyroid artery and recurrent laryngeal nerve [1, 2, 5], almost at the level of the cricoid cartilage. True ectopies of normal glands are rarely major and the glands are lateral to the cricoid cartilage, latero-pharyngeal or inter-crico-thyroideal in 12 to 13% of cases. In less than 1% of cases, the superior glands are above the upper pole of the thyroid lobe. True retropharyngeal and retro esophageal positions are found in 1 to 4% of cases [1, 7, 8]. Figure 1.2. shows the result of superior parathyroid location in a Swedish Autopsy series from the 1980s [4]. Abnormally enlarged superior glands may migrate caudally nearer to the inferior glands or even more distantly into the posterior mediastinum [9] as shown in figure 1.3. However, they remain posterior to the thyroid lobe with a vascular origin supero-posteror to the recurrent laryngeal nerve. This can be a major cause of repeated failures to cure primary hyperparathyroidism, when this posterior relationship of the superior gland is not understood leading to less experienced surgeons mistaking superior for inferior glands and vice versa.

In contrast, the final resting position of non-pathologic inferior parathyroid glands is much wider than the superior glands and extends from the Parapharyngeal skull base to the pericardium [10]. Figure 1.4. shows the location of the inferior parathyroid glands based on the Swedish autopsy series [4]. The inferior parathyroid is nearly always anterior to the recurrent laryngeal nerve. In 61% of cases, parathyroids are located at the level of the inferior thyroid pole in this anterior plane [11]. In 26 to 39% of cases, they are within the thyrothymic ligament or the superior cervical thymic part [2, 8, 11]. Less frequently, in 7%, they are positioned more cephalad, close to the superior glands with which they can be confused if the pedicles relationship to the recurrent laryngeal nerve is not appreciated as described above.

An ectopic position superior to the superior parathyroid glands or within the carotid sheath only occurs in less than 1 to 2% [1, 2, 12] while low positions in the chest outside of the thymic tissue are also rare affecting 1-2% with parathyroid glands located in the superior, anterior or posterior mediastinum or the aorto-pulmonary window of the middle mediastinum [1]. Despite these considerable topographic variations, parathyroid gland arrangements are symmetric in both sides of the neck in 80%, superior glands being a little more symmetric than the inferiors, 80% and 70%, respectively [5, 13]. Intra-thyroid localization of parathyroid tissue in autopsy specimens was 0.2% [5] whilst others have reported higher incidences upto 3.5% in selected groups [1, 5, 14-16]. However, the incidence of intra-thyroid glands is more frequent in re-operative disease. The number of parathyroid glands is four in 84% of the general population [5]. The inferior parathyroid gland is usually anterior to the recurrent laryngeal nerve while the superior gland is always posterior to it [1, 5, 10, 18]. While 6 to 13% of persons have super-nummary parathyroid glands less than 4 glands are rarely found [5, 10, 17] and those cases reported may be due to missed glands. Supernumerary glands can occupy rare, yet exceptional ectopic cervical or mediastinal localizations such as the middle mediastinum, the aorto-pulmonary window or the carotid sheath as outlined in the embryology section [1,19,20]. Normal parathyroid glands are mellow supple, well-encapsulated smooth structures frequently surrounded by fat. Older studies have described normal mean dimensions varying from 5 x 3 x 1 mm to 8.3 x 4.4 x 1.8 mm for an average weight of 40 mg per gland (extremes: 10 to 78 mg) [7, 11]. A recent study of parathyroid gland size and volume in relation to vitamin D status has shown that while vitamin D deficiency causes hyperplasia the median gland volume in those that are not vitamin D deficient was $25mm^3$[21].

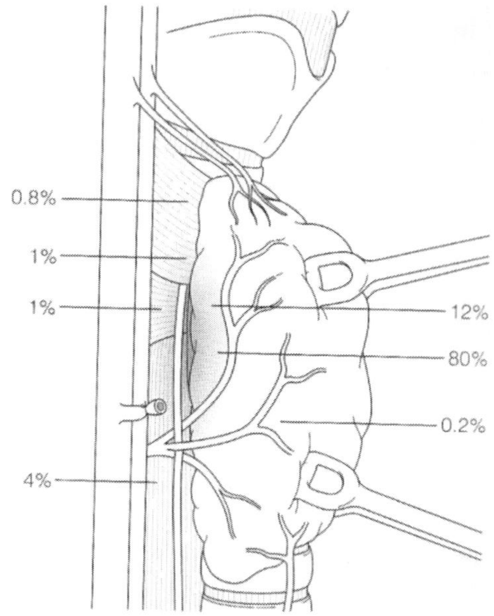

Figure 1.2. Superior parathyroid gland positions based on the result of 503 autopsies. This article was published in Surgery, 95, Akerstrom G, Malmaeus J, Bergstrom R, Surgical anatomy of human parathyroid glands, 14-21, Copyright Elsevier 1984.

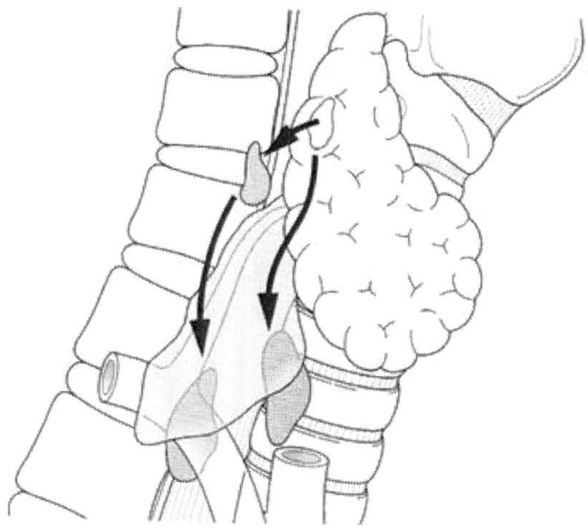

Figure 1.3. Migratory path of enlarged superior parathyroid glands. They tend to migrate inferiorly and posteriorly so that surgeons unfamiliar with the unchanging relationship of the pedicle to the RLN can mistake superior for inferior glands. This article was published in Surgery of the thyroid and parathyroid glands, Randolph GW, Urken ML, 507-28, Copyright Elsevier 2003.

Their surface is shiny and their color is creamy brown. They are often surrounded by fat but a sliding movement of a slightly darker area within the fatty tissue is almost pathognomic of the parathyroid gland. Different shapes are described varying from round to rod-like form [7].

Parathyroid Glands Vascularization

Anatomical studies [21,22] have shown that arterial blood supply of 80 to 86% of superior parathyroid glands and 90 to 95% of inferior parathyroids comes from branches of the inferior thyroid artery. The vascularization of inferior parathyroid glands depends primarily on the inferior thyroid artery. The inferior thyroid artery also supplies the superior parathyroid glands in 85%, and by the posterior branch of the superior thyroid artery, or by the posterior marginal arch of Evans in the rest. Therefore both the inferior and superior parathyroid glands may be entirely dependent on the inferior thyroid artery. For some authors, the inferior thyroid artery exclusively irrigates the four parathyroid glands in 85% of the general population [1]. Studies comparing hypoparathyroidism in central ligation of the inferior thyroid artery versus capsular dissection showed that capsular dissection avoided hypoparathyroidism [24][25]. For others, the contribution of the superior thyroid artery is not negligible. Nies et al. [23] showed through a randomized study that ligation of the inferior thyroid artery trunk does not increase the risk of hypoparathyroidism after bilateral subtotal thyroidectomy. The low rate of hypoparathyroidism after ligation of the four thyroid arteries was reported by Johansson et al [24] in the specific setting of bilateral subtotal thyroidectomy without dissection of the posterior thyroid lobe. Delivery of arterial blood to parathyroids was thought to be guaranteed by anastomotic branches of pharyngeal, laryngeal, tracheal, esophageal and bronchial arteries with the inferior and superior thyroid arteries. Additionally, based on a Laser-Doppler fluometry of 53 parathyroid glands in 45 patients with thyroid or parathyroid disease, the authors concluded that blood supply of parathyroid glands is not limited to the inferior thyroid arteries but that other sources may also contribute such as the superior thyroid artery, the thyrothymic cord, arteries of the connective tissue between thyroid and parathyroid glands and isthmic anastomoses between bilateral thyroid arteries. Finally, on a dissection of 52 cadavers, Nobori et al. [21] found that the superior thyroid artery almost always irrigates the superior parathyroid glands in addition to supply from the inferior ones.

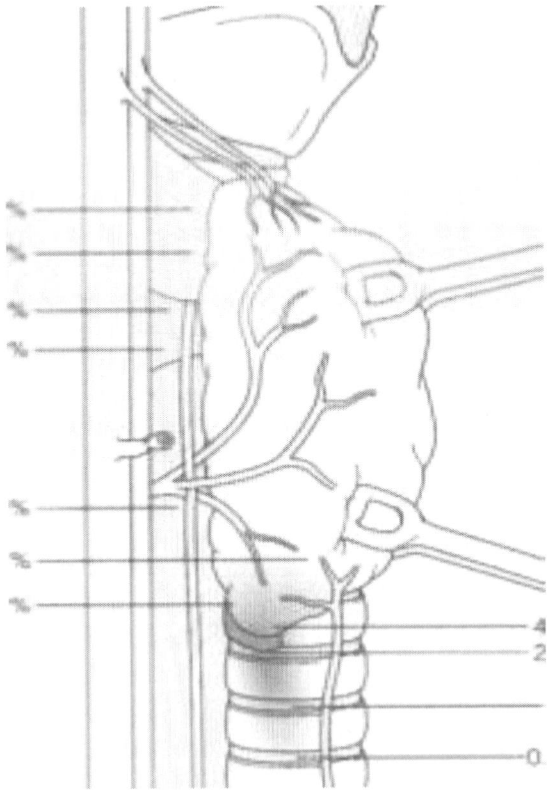

Figure 1.4. Inferior parathyroid gland positions based on the result of 503 autopsies. This article was published in Surgery, 95, Akerstrom G, Malmaeus J, Bergstrom R, Surgical anatomy of human parathyroid glands, 14-21, Copyright Elsevier 1984.

Regardless of whether one believes the inferior or branches of the superior thyroid artery supply the superior glands a capsular dissection technique in thyroidectomy will safe guard either and has become the procedure of choice. It is probably most important to note that these studies were done in sub-total thyroidectomy, which no longer has a place since total thyroidectomy became the operation of choice in graves disease. Careful capsular dissection of the thyroid with identification and preservation of parathyroid vasculature is what prevents hypoparathyroidism rather than whether it ultimately originates from the superior or inferior thyroid artery as has been shown [24, 25]. Parathyroid glands located in the thyrothymic ligament or in the upper portion of the thymus are dependent on the inferior thyroid arteries whereas mediastinal glands may be supplied by the internal mammary artery, a thymic artery or more rarely by a branch from the aorta [1, 11]. The arterial supply of the parathyroid glands is terminal in type; the artery is solitary in two thirds of cases. The length of each artery can vary from 1 to 40 mm [1, 13], but in cases of thyroidectomy, even if the parathyroid is pedicled, its preservation depends primarily on the distance between the origin of its artery and the thyroid capsule. Therefore, during thyroid lobectomy, the inferior thyroid artery must never be ligated centrally, at the level of its main trunk. Similarly, the preservation of superior parathyroid requires separate ligation of the branches of the superior thyroid artery so as to preserve the posterior branch and or anastomotic branches that may supply the superior gland. Venous drainage of parathyroid glands occurs by three methods: 1)-by the capsular network of the thyroid, 2)- by the venous pedicles of the thyroid body, or 3)-by combination [1,11]. Thyroid lobectomy may render the ipsilateral parathyroid glands ischemic. Haemostasis of a parathyroid vein generally should be avoided but probably doesn't lead to permanent hypoparathyroidism. Damage to the arterial supply of the parathyroid causes the gland to lighten in colour and become pale, this represents permanent dysfunction of that gland. Parathyroid ischemia due to venous damge causes congestion evidenced by progressive darkening of the gland and may predict impending dysfunction. When a subcapsular parathyroid haematoma occurs incision of the capsule and superficial parenchymareleases the haematoma and allows the gland to recover its normal color s. [1,2].

Conclusion

- Knowledge of embryology and anatomy are mandatory for thyroid and parathyroid surgery if it is to be done with low morbidity.
- The arterial supply of the parathyroid glands is terminal in type.
- The vascularization of inferior and superior parathyroids depends primarily on the inferior thyroid artery. However, the inferior thyroid artery also supplies 15% of superior parathyroids, by the posterior branch of the superior thyroid artery, or by the posterior marginal arch of Evans.
- During thyroidectomy, the preservation of parathyroid glands is ensured by the capsular dissection technique.
- Parathyroid glands drainage may reach one of the three thyroid veins or the venous complex along the thyroid capsule.

References

[1] Henry, JF; Denizot, A. Bases anatomiques et embryologiques de l'hyperparathyroïd-isme primaire. In: *L'hyperparathyroïdisme primaire*. Paris: Springer-Verlag; 1991; 5-14.

[2] Fancy, T; Gallagher, D 3rd; Hornig, JD. Surgical anatomy of the thyroid and parathyroid glands. *Otolaryngol Clin. North Am,* 2010 43, 221-227.

[3] Henry, JF. Title: Surgical Anatomy and Embryology of the Thyroid and Parathyroid Glands and Recurrent and External Laryngeal Nerves. In: Elsevier. *Title: Textbook of Endocrine Surgery.* Saunders; 2006; 9-15.

[4] Akerstrom, G; Malmaeus, J; Bergstrom, R. Surgical anatomy of human parathyroid glands. *Surgery,* 1984 95, 14-21.

[5] Mansberger, AR Jr; Wei, JP. Surgical embryology and anatomy of the thyroid and parathyroid glands. *Surg. Clin. North Am,* 1993 73, 727-746.
[6] Chevallier, JM; Martelli, H; Wind, P. [Surgical discovery of parathyroid glands and the recurrent laryngeal nerve. Application of well known embryological concepts in the operating room]. *Ann. Chir,* 1995 49, 296-304.
[7] Wang, C. The anatomic basis of parathyroid surgery. *Ann. Surg,* 1976 183, 271-275.
[8] Nanka, O; Sedý, J; Vítková, I; Libánský, P; Adámek, S. Surgical anatomy of parathyroid glands with emphasis on parathyroidectomy. *Prague Med. Rep,* 2006 107, 261-272.
[9] Phitayakorn, R; McHenry, CR. Incidence and location of ectopic abnormal parathyroid glands. *Am. J. Surg,* 2006 191, 418-423.
[10] Geeta, L; Clark,OH. Title: Thyroid, Parathyroid and Adrenal. In: Mc-Graw-Hill. *Title: Schwartz's Principles of Surgery.* 2005; 1395-1470.
[11] Abboud, B. [Topographic anatomy and arterial vascularization of the parathyroid glands. Practical application]. *Presse Med,* 1996 25, 1156-1161.
[12] Billingsley, KG; Fraker, DL; Doppman, JL; Norton, JA; Shawker, TH; Skarulis, MC; Marx, SJ; Spiegel, AM; Alexander, HR. Localization and operative management of undescended parathyroid adenomas in patients with persistent primary hyperpara-thyroidism. *Surgery,* 1994 116, 982-989.
[13] Bliss, RD; Gauger, PG; Delbridge, LW. Surgeon's approach to the thyroid gland: surgical anatomy and the importance of technique. *World J. Surg,* 2000 24, 891-897.
[14] Sarfati, E; De Ferron, P; Gossot, D; Assens, P; Dubost, C. [Parathyroid adenoma at an atypical site, ectopic or not]. *J. Chir. (Paris),* 1987 124, 24-29.
[15] Proye, C; Bizard, JP; Carnaille, B; Quiévreux, JL. [Hyperparathyroidism and intrathyroid parathyroid gland. 43 cases]. *Ann. Chir,* 1994 48, 501-506.
[16] Abboud, B; Sleilaty, G; Ayoub, S; Hachem, K; Smayra, T; Ghorra, C; Abadjian, G. Intrathyroid parathyroid adenoma in primary hyperparathyroidism: can it be predicted preoperatively? *World J. Surg,* 2007 31, 817-823.
[17] Delattre, JF; Flament, JB; Palot, JP; Pluot, M. [Variations in the parathyroid glands. Number, situation and arterial vascularization. Anatomical study and surgical application]. *J. Chir. (Paris),* 1982 119, 633-641.
[18] Gilmour, JR: The gross anatomy of the parathyroid glands. *J. Pathol,* 1938 46:133.
[19] Prinz, RA; Lonchyna, V; Carnaille, B; Wurtz, A; Proye, C. Thoracoscopic excision of enlarged mediastinal parathyroid glands. *Surgery,* 1994 116, 999-1004.
[20] Deleplanque, G; Kraimps, JL; Coste, G; Carretier, M; Barbier, J. [A case of parathyroid adenoma localized in the middle mediastinum]. *Ann. Chir,* 1989 43, 393-396.
[21] Kirkby-Bott J, El-Khatib Z, Soudan B, Caiazzo R, Arnalsteen L, Carnaille B. 25 hydroxy vitamin D deficiency causes parathyroid incidentalomas. *Langenbeck Arch. Surg,*2010; 395:919-924.
[22] Nobori, M; Saiki, S; Tanaka, N; Harihara, Y; Shindo, S; Fujimoto, Y. Blood supply of the parathyroid gland from the superior thyroid artery. *Surgery,* 1994 115, 417–423.
[23] Flament, JB; Delattre, JF; Pluot, M. Arterial blood supply of the parathyroid glands; implications for thyroid surgery. *Anat. Clin,* 1982 3, 279-287.

[24] Thomusch O, Machens A, Sekulla C, Ukkat J, Lippert H, Gastinger I, Dralle H. Multivariate analysis of risk factors for postoperative complications in benign goiter surgery: Prospective multicenter study in germany. *World J. Surg.* 2000;24(11):1335-41.

[25] Thomusch O, Machens A, Sekulla C, Ukkat J, Brauckhoff M, Dralle H. The impact of surgical technique on postoperative hypoparathyroidism in bilateral thyroid surgery: A multivariate analysis of 5846 consecutive patients. *Surgery* 2003;133(2):180-5.

[26] Nies, C; Sitter, H; Zielke, A; Bandorski, T; Menze, J; Ehlenz, K; Rothmund, M. Parathyroid function following ligation of the inferior thyroid arteries during bilateral subtotal thyroidectomy. *Br. J. Surg,* 1994 81, 1757-1759.

[27] Johansson, K; Ander, S; Lennquist, S; Smeds, S. Human parathyroid blood supply determined by laser-Doppler flowmetry. *World J. Surg,* 1994 18, 417-420.

In: Parathyroid: Anatomy, Functions and Disorders
Editor: James Kirkby-Bott
ISBN: 978-1-62100-765-4

Chapter II

Imaging of the Parathyroid Glands

Yassar A. Qureshi, Colin Todd, and James Kirkby-Bott
Kingston Hospital, Surrey, UK

Introduction

The purpose of imaging of the parathyroid glands is mainly for localisation of the abnormal gland(s) and pre-operative surgical planning. A number of imaging modalities are available, each with its own indications, advantages and disadvantages. However, given that surgical intervention is still the treatment of most parathyroid diseases and that minimally invasive surgery in localised primary hyperparathyroidism is becoming the gold standard, the importance of imaging takes on a paramount value: to avoid unsuccessful explorative surgery.

Normal parathyroid glands are not normally seen on most imaging modalities, given that their mean size is 6x4x2mm[1,2]. However, in the diseased state, be that an adenoma, carcinoma or hyperplasia, the glands become distinct from their surrounding structures, and can be identified more readily. Further, of the four parathyroid glands - two superior and particularly the two inferior, ectopic locations are not uncommon. As part of pre-operative planning it is essential that ectopic glands are identified, and the newer imaging modalities can identify such glands quite accurately. The ectopic location may be as diverse as the retro-oesophageal space, the mediastinum, or even the skull base as described in chapter 1. Also, 5% of patients may have supernumerary glands, and both clinician and radiologist should be alert to this [3,4]. Importantly, it is useful to remember that imaging forms only a part of the investigative and management process that is essential to treat parathyroid disease. Clinical and family history, biochemical studies and imaging all contribute to the development of a diagnosis, which allows the endocrinologist or surgeon to ably treat these diseases. Whilst ultrasound and sestamibi are routinely used in localisation other modalities are increasing interest, particularly when ultrasound and sestamibi have been unable to localise the diseased gland. The purpose of this chapter is to describe the main imaging techniques available for the assessment of diseased parathyroid glands, or as part of investigation into deranged biochemical function. The uses, indications, advantages and pitfalls of each modality are discussed.

Ultrasonography (US)

Ultrasound scanning is one of 2 modalities (sestamibi and ultrasound) routinely used to image the parathyroid glands. It is usually the first radiological imaging performed once disease of the parathyroid has been biochemically proven. The reason for this is not only its accuracy but also its convenience, ease of use and low cost. However, it is user dependent, and hence has a variable sensitivity and specificity, and may not always give the conclusive answer that both clinician and patient yearn. In experienced hands the sensitivity and specificity are excellent. US utilises the conversion of sound energy into a visual image, based on the Doppler principle. Essentially, an ultrasound machine generates an ultrasonic pulse at very high frequency, typically greater than 10 Mhz, which reflects off structures it comes into contact with. Thus, differing wavelengths of energy are returned based on the depth of contact, and also the consistency of the structure being examined. A real-time three-dimensional image is constructed using this information, and the experienced sonographer will be able to make conclusions as to the state of the structure being imaged. Both grey scale and colour Doppler can be utilised, the latter being particularly useful to assess the vascularity of diseased glands [5]. The patient is examined in the supine position with the neck extended, thereby making the depth of the neck to be examined relatively shorter. The parathyroids can be visualised and contrasted to the surrounding thyroid tissue, which is of differing sonographic character. The main diagnoses that can be established at sonography include a parathyroid adenoma, which accounts for the vast majority of diseased glands, hyperplasia, or even a carcinoma. An adenoma invariably manifests as an enlarged gland, and on scanning are almost always homogenous in appearance (figure 2.1). Although they are usually smooth and round, they may be multi-lobulated and will appear as a discrete mass when compared to surrounding tissue [6]. A feeding vessel is often seen, and this gives a characteristic vascular rim around the adenoma (figure 2.2) [7,8]. Once a single adenoma has been visualised, it is essential that the remaining parathyroids are examined too, as double or multiple adenomas usually manifest synchronously [4]. A hyperplastic gland is normally smaller than an adenoma, thus making it difficult to identify [9]. The principle method of identification refers to its hypoechogenicity compared to surrounding thyroid tissue. Parathyroid carcinomas have a distinct appearance of variable echogenicity, with rough edges and a bulky capsule, with most displaying hypervascularity. However, they represent 1% of parathyroid disease [10]· There are no studies that have tried to distinguish atypical adenomas from typical adenomas or carcinoma (figure 2.3).

Ectopic glands are often difficult to identify on ultrasonography with confidence, particularly if they are intra-thyroid or mediastinal. Compression of surrounding tissues to elicit a parathyroid can be utilised, but now other modalities are used in conjunction with far more accurate localisations [5]. Also, diseased thyroid tissue, particularly inflammatory conditions and multi-nodular goitre, can make visualisation of the parathyroids extremely difficult, even for the experienced sonographer [11,12].

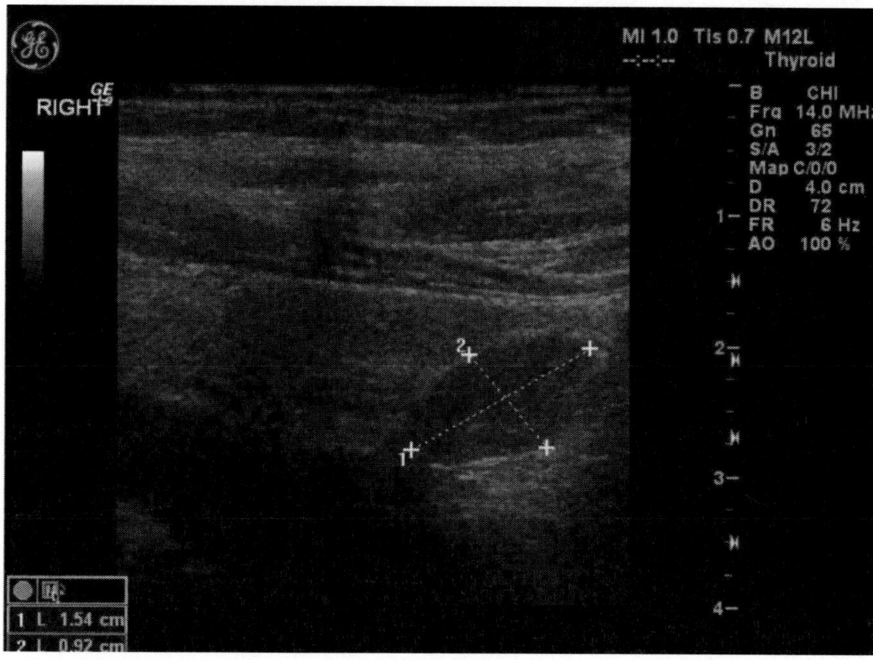

Figure 2.1. Shows the homogenous appearance of a parathyroid adenoma and its hypoechogenicity.

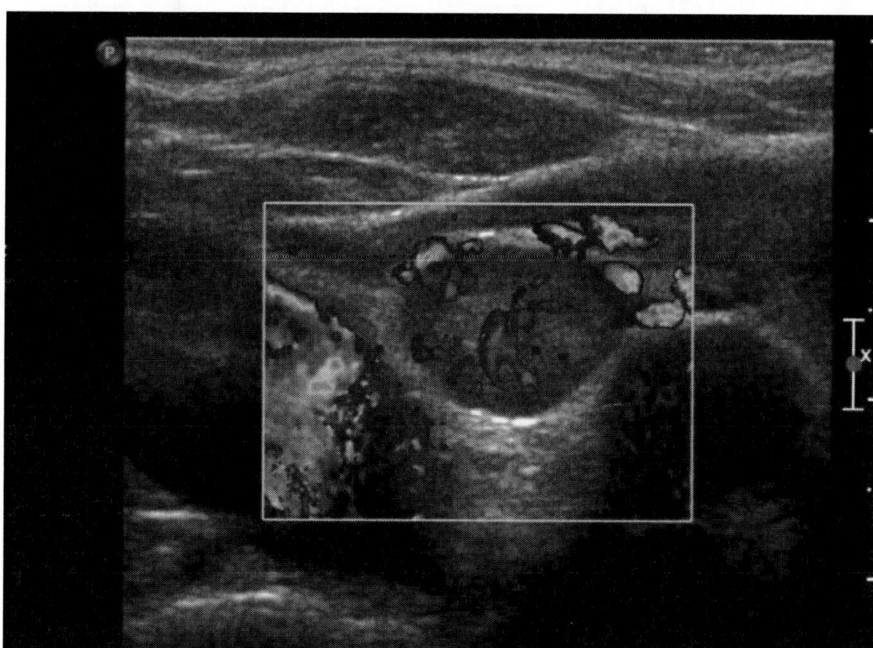

Figure 2.2. Shows the vascular rim seen around parathyroid adenomas with Doppler.

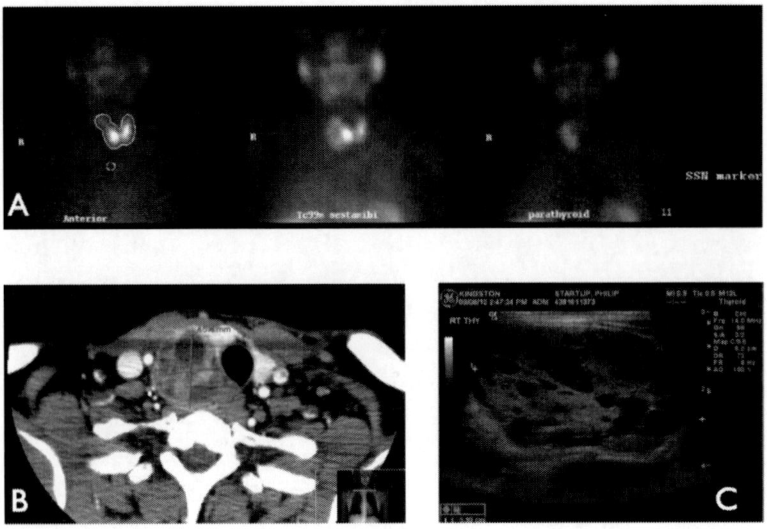

Figure 2.3. A. Sestamibi of the parathyroid carcinoma seen in B and C images. B. CT imaging of a large parathyroid cancer showing its heterogeneous appearance, C. US of parathyroid cancer also appearing large and heterogeneous compared to the adenoma shown in figure 2.1.

Ultrasound could potentially be of use in pre-operative diagnosis due to its use in performing guided fine needle aspiration. Several papers documenting the use of FNA techniques to get tissue to perform PTH assay analysis on have been described in the intra-operative setting, but not pre-operatively [13-17]. Further, suspicious thyroid nodules may be cytologically examined synchronously. However, the main established use of ultrasound is in pre-operative marking of a diseased gland. This can assist the surgeon to perform a focused operation to excise the disease gland, and avoids the need for more extensive dissection. The sensitivities of pre-operative marking using ultrasound range from 72% to 89% for adenomas; indicating the user-dependent nature of the examination [18,19]. The highest sensitivities are for adenomas, which are distinct, but much lower for hyperplastic glands at 40-50%. Carcinomas are detected with a sensitivity of 50-90%[12,20]. More recently, ethanol ablation of parathyroid glands has been used to treat patients with primary hyperparathyroidism. Ethanol is injected directly into the gland under sonographic guidance, until its vascular supply is diminished. Such a technique is particularly useful in the pre-morbid patient, but has been associated with local pain and dysphonia when used to treat thyroid nodules [21]. Rare parathyroid cysts can also be drained with an FNAC needle under US guidance. They seldom recur and the cyst fluid can be used to confirm the diagnosis. Ultrasound is of most use when used in conjunction with Sestamibi scanning. Concordant imaging is much more specific than unimodality imaging. The success rate of minimally invasive parathyroidectomy in this setting is successful in 98% of patients compared to 90-95% in unimodality imaging [19]

Nuclear Medicine Imaging

The use of radiotracers for scanning the parathyroids has reached great prominence over the last few years, in a large part due to the comparatively superior sensitivity, specificity and overall accuracy of these studies. Further, in contrast to ultrasound, it is a relatively user-independent procedure. The most frequently used nuclear medicine test for imaging the parathyroids in the setting of primary hyperparathyroidism is sestamibi Technetium (^{99m}Tc) scintigraphy [6]. This radioisotope is taken up avidly by the hyperfunctioning parathyroid tissue, and hence can be readily located on imaging. Sestamibi ^{99m}Tc is a single radiotracer study. The problem with such single tracer studies is that uptake is not tissue specific. In this case, the radiotracer is taken up by both thyroid and parathyroid tissue, but the reason for its particular use is that hyperfunctioning parathyroid glands will avidly uptake the radiotracer quicker, and will retain it for longer. Therefore, early images will show such parathyroids as having a denser uptake than surrounding tissues, and delayed, washout, images will still show retained radiotracer avidity after 2 hours. Dual radiotracer, or subtraction, techniques are also often used. This involves the injection of both sestamibi ^{99m}Tc and a second agent, mostly pertechnetate ^{99m}Tc or ^{123}I sodium iodide. The thyroid takes up the latter agents only, and the contrast between the radiotracer uptakes can thus be compared more effectively to identify parathyroid glands [23]. Indeed, ectopic parathyroids can be identified in this manner too, based on their pattern of uptake. Needless to say, the patient is again examined in the supine position with the head in slight extension. Sestamibi ^{99m}Tc radiotracer is injected intravenously. A second radiotracer, for subtraction testing, can be intravenously administered after the first injection. After a delay of 5-15 minutes, images are taken, mostly only in planar views, using a range of techniques (figure 2.4). Single photon emission computed tomography (SPECT) or SPECT with CT might be used [24]. After 2-3 hours, delayed images are taken. Depending on the camera used, images can be reconstructed in a number of planes. The principle behind radioisotope nuclear imaging lies in the ability of different tissues to take up the radiotracer, based on their metabolism and kinetics. The ability of the scan to identify diseased parathyroids is based on the fact that such glands have reduced clearance of the tracer over time. Such subtleties can lead to minor changes in the gland to be detected on imaging. Differing tracers work in different ways, and sestamibi works as a blood flow tracer, hence is particularly useful in detecting adenomas with their characteristic vascularity. A large meta-analysis incorporating 96 studies in the use of sestamibi ^{99m}Tc found an overall sensitivity of 88% for detecting solitary adenomas when used for investigating primary hyperparathyroidism [25]. Another large series reported sensitivity of 90% in detection of single adenomas, 73% for multiple adenomas and 45% for hyperplasia [26]. These were studies where sestamibi ^{99m}Tc was used as a solitary investigation method pre-operatively for localisation, and reveal a slight improvement when compared to the traditional method of ultrasound.

The method of assessing the imaging relates to comparison of the thyroid with surrounding tissue, both on immediate and delayed images. Any initial increased activity and focal activity persisting on delayed images is suggestive of a parathyroid adenoma. The images are assessed in the typical locations of where parathyroid glands are located, but also in ectopic locations, where similar avid-behaviour will differentiate the glands from other structures, such as lymph nodes. Often, either the immediate or delayed images will be equivocal, but often typical uptake behaviour in one is sufficient for a diagnosis where there is clinical concern. There are some difficulties that are encountered with the use of nuclear imaging. Most significantly, there is no radioisotope that is specific for the parathyroid gland, either normal or diseased. Thus, a combination of factors is required to be met to detect these glands, including, most importantly, that there is no abnormal uptake in surrounding tissue.

For example, thyroid adenomas and carcinomas, especially of the Hürthle cell variety, very closely mimic the behaviour of parathyroid adenomas [27].

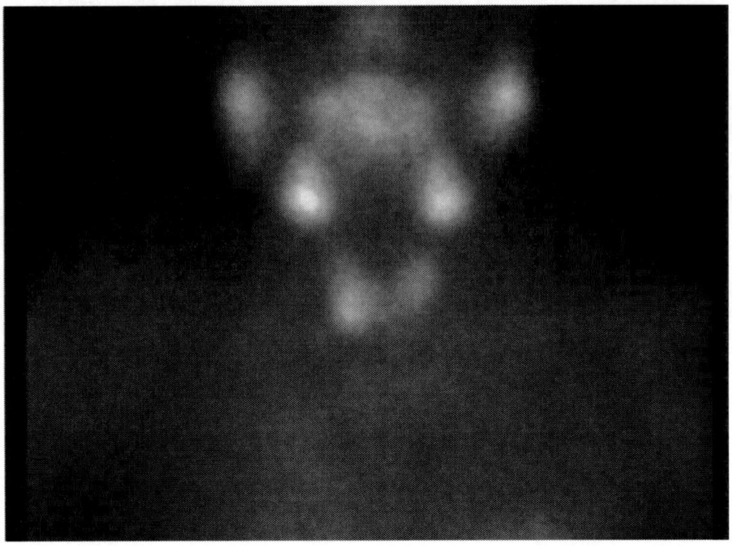

Figure 2.4. Sestamibi scan after 15mins washout time showing persistence of radiotracer on the right hand side. US is needed to confirm whether it is likely to be an inferior gland or migrated superior gland.

Similarly, inflammatory conditions affecting the thyroid or other neck structures can cause such a heterogeneous uptake that parathyroid avidity is masked. However, newer techniques in image display, such as SPECT-CT, are being employed to somewhat useful effect to negate this problem.[24] Levels of plasma 25-hydroxyvitamin D are thought to have a relationship with the severity of hyperparathyroidism. Generally, it is thought that the lower the serum vitamin D concentration, the more severe the parathyroid hyperplasia and this is also particularly true for adenoma. With respect to sestamibi nuclear imaging, an intriguing association between low serum vitamin D and detection of adenomas is thought to exist. Essentially, low vitamin D results has a higher sensitivity of detecting adenomas by sestamibi, and this is thought to relate to increased rates of bone turn over, and possibly by nurturing more aggressive adenoma [28]. However, another explanation may be that calcium levels are more dependent upon parathyroid activity in vitamin D deficiency based on the physiological model described by Kirkby-Bott *et al* in relation to postoperative hypo-calcaemia [29]. These hyper-functioning and larger adenomas are subsequently detected by scanning more readily. Positron Emission Tomography (PET) is another nuclear medicine technique that is finding greater application all the time, particularly as a staging tool, and as a means to detect occult disease. It works on a similar principle, in that a radiotracer, for example ^{11}C Methionine, or FDG is taken up by tissue, and varying rates of metabolism and kinetics give rise to a particular pattern of uptake detected on images. However, it is still not in widespread use specifically to assess primary or recurrent hyperparathyroidism, but its use is gaining popularity, owing to its reported superior sensitivity [30,31]. Sensitivity of 100% and specificity of 88.9% have been recently reported [32] The importance of nuclear imaging, especially of sestamibi, has been further validated by large studies assessing the use of combined modalities, that is to say sestamibi ^{99}Tc scintigraphy and ultrasonography.

The sensitivities of both techniques combined, as opposed to each as a solitary investigation, appear to be much higher in locating diseased glands. Studies have shown a successful location based on combined use of both modalities as high as 95%, although the range usually lies between 79% and 90%[18,33,34]. Using both techniques allows both the detection of normally placed glands and ectopics, with each modality providing different, but complementary, information. The importance of minimal access surgery has gained such popularity that combined imaging techniques are now becoming quite the norm in many centres. A successful pre-operative localisation results in the higher chance of more focused, limited surgery.

Computerised Tomography (CT)

CT scanning in the context of parathyroid disease is less frequently utilised, bar a few circumstances where it is important for optimal patient management. It is often used in conjunction with other investigations, particularly nuclear medicine techniques. The high-resolution images, with added contrast, are also of great benefit in preoperative surgical planning.

The main use of CT is where ultrasonography has failed in the identification of a diseased parathyroid gland. This may be the case if it lies in an ectopic position, or if patient habitus or multinodular thyroid goitre makes the use of ultrasound particularly difficult. It is also useful in assessing recurrent cases of hyperparathyroidism. However, the greatest use of CT is reserved for cases of parathyroid adenocarcinoma, for a multitude of reasons. Firstly, it is used to assess the degree of local invasion, as well as the primary characteristics of the malignant tumour. Knowledge of proximity to surrounding vital structures is essential prior to surgical intervention. Secondly, it is used as a staging tool, as for any other malignancy.

CT images are obtained with the use of high dose X-ray radiation, which is circumferentially emitted around the patient. Sensors detect the X-rays once they have dissipated through the object, and this information is relayed to a computerised system that reconstructs this information as images. These are formatted as 3-dimensional views, and allow volumetric reconstruction to be performed. Various scanners work in slightly differing ways, and pictures obtained are taken anywhere between 1.25mm to 5mm apart. This gives, particularly the former, a very high degree of detail. Images can be deciphered in a number of planes; the most commonly used one being axial. In addition, intravenous contrast media can be used, thus highlighting certain targets and making the reading of scans even more useful. Currently, triple-phase scans can be performed, where images are taken pre-, peri- and post-contrast, allowing a highly detailed examination of the vasculature of subject tissue [36]. The scan is performed with the patient in a supine position, again with the neck slightly extended. The area to be scanned varies, but generally includes the skull base and extends inferiorly to include the mediastinum and chest. Parathyroids increase their signal density 45-70 seconds post contrast and then lose it whereas lymph nodes retain signal and gain it less quickly. These timed scans are known as 4D CT and by using 1.5mm slices they have higher sensitivity and specificity than conventional CT scanning [36]. This technique can also be used with SPECT as described in the section on nuclear medicine. CT scans remain time consuming and relatively costly, but by far their biggest drawback is the use of high dose radiation. Although not considered a problem, regular and repeated use of CT scans is thought to be associated with the development of some malignancies, and thus should be avoided. However, the detail that is obtained from CT images is often necessary such that the benefits outweigh the potential risk. Thyroid pathology needs to be excluded using USS +/- FNAC before CT scanning so that iodine contrast used in the parathyroid scan doesn't complicate thyroid cancer treatment if thyroid cancer pathology is also present. In the context of parathyroid disease, CT scanning with contrast is particularly useful. Parathyroid adenomas, although non-specific in appearance on CT, are typically vascular, and contrast scans may reveal a small 1-2cm mass either in a normal or ectopic position with rapid uptake. This feature allows identification of parathyroid adenomas, and hyperplasia, especially when compared to local structures of a similar appearance, such as regional lymph nodes. The uptake of contrast reflects the vascularity, and appears swifter than other structures in the neck [5,35]. The sensitivity for detecting abnormal parathyroid glands using CT alone ranges from 46% to 87%[36]. CT scanning is becoming a necessary adjunct in assessing suspected cases of malignancy. This is true for both primary and recurrent disease, as it will guide intervention. Seldom, however, a complex adenoma or parathyroid cyst may produce puzzling images which may be interpreted as a malignant tumour, thus reinforcing the need for concurrent imaging, be that an ultrasound scan or nuclear imaging. CT is also of great use when sestamibi localises disease outside of the neck, particularly in the mediastinum where ultrasound is not reliable. Depending upon the more detailed anatomical location seen on CT, guided by the sestamibi result, different locations in the neck can influence surgical approach, as thoracoscopy, mediastinoscopy and sternal/manubrial split are all possibilities. The major issue with CT scanning is that small adenomas or hyperplastic glands can be difficult to detect, given the number of similar sized structures in the head and neck. The non-specific features of such soft tissue masses are often difficult to conclusively infer an opinion on. However, as mentioned, with added intravenous contrast, such decipherment may be made far more readily. Newer CT techniques, such as 4-dimensional imaging are being increasingly utilised for head and neck scanning. Some studies report sensitivities of up to 88% for such techniques when localising hyper-functioning parathyroid glands. However, even when assessing for local relapse of parathyroid malignancy, sensitivity of standard CT may be as low as 53%[37]. It is for these reasons that CT is seldom used as a solitary radiological investigation, although it still maintains some value in selected cases.

Magnetic Resonance Imaging (MRI)

The indications for MRI in the context of parathyroid disease are similar to those for the use of CT. Thus, MRI is used largely as an adjunct rather than a solitary investigation. It fulfils the requirement of sometimes identifying ectopic adenomas where ultrasonography has failed, and has uses in the assessment of primary and recurrent malignancy, as well as in refractory hyperparathyroidism [38]. MRI utilises a strong magnetic field to align hydrogen atoms in the body. A radiofrequency transmitter that is built into the scanner generates such a strong field. As the alignment of magnetisation shifts, the atoms produce a characteristic rotational field. However, as the magnetic field shifts away, the atoms revert to their original state. The energy difference between the changes is detected as photons are emitted. This subtle change is detected by the scanner, and can be used to construct a view of the body. Images are typically viewed in 3-dimension. Different tissues have differing atomic composition, and it is these differences that allow excellent delineation between structures. Images are registered as either T1 or T2, dependent on the water content and fat suppression of the tissues being assessed. Intravenous contrast in the form of gadolinium is often used to further enhance the contrast resolution of MRI scanning. Similar to CT, the patient is examined supine with the neck slightly extended. Given the superior tissue contrast that MRI offers in comparison to CT, it is reserved for difficult cases. This is particularly the case for ectopic glands, especially if affected by hyperplasia or adenoma [38]. Typically, they appear as enhancing masses, with increased signal on T2 images, and lower intensity of T1 images [5]. However, up to 40% of abnormal parathyroid glands lack this uptake signal, so their identification is dependent on knowledge of normal or ectopic location [39,40]. Indeed, local lymph nodes have similar appearances to parathyroid tissue on MRI. As with CT, MRI is useful at assessing the local advancement of primary carcinoma, or to gauge recurrent disease. It may be particularly useful when seeking abnormal regional lymph nodes, which contain metastases. The distinct advantage of MRI scanning lies in the absence of any radiation, and its better tissue contrast compared to CT. However, parathyroid glands, diseased and normal, are often difficult to detect. This is made worse when there is concomitant thyroid disease. Further, given that the examination process is extremely sensitive, even slight movement can alter the final images; artefacts further making decipherment difficult. Again, MRI has a role to play in imaging of the parathyroids, but similar to CT, it is limited as an adjunct rather than a solitary investigation.

Table 2.1. Overview of imaging modalities in parathyroid disease

Imaging Modality	Sensitivity (%)	Specificity (%)	False Positives(%)	Advantages	Disadvantages
Ultrasound*	72-89	80	15-20	Inexpensive. No ionising radiation. Can combine with FNA techniques.	Operator dependant. Difficult with ectopic positions.
Technectium - Sestamibi scan*	88 overall 90 single, 73 multiple, 45 hyperplasia	98	<3	CT-SPECT offers better localisation. Best method available minimal radiation.	False negatives in multi-gland disease.
CT scan + iv contrast	46-70	80	50	4-D CT has much better localisation	Ionising radiation and i.v contrast needed.
MRI scan	64-85	88-95	18	Good at localising ectopic glands	Expensive. Claustrophobic

*Concordant sestamibi and US results have a sensitivity 95% and accuracy of 91%.

Conclusion

Although each technique offers its own advantages and disadvantages (Table 2.1), the mainstay of radiological diagnosis for hyperparathyroidism currently is ultrasound and sestamibi ^{99m}Tc scintigraphy. The combination of these two investigations has allowed a greater deal of sensitivity than any other combination or with any modality on its own. CT has a role where sestamibi localises disease outside the neck beyond the reach of ultrasound, such as the mediastinum where more accurate localisation can influence the surgical approach.

The reason for imaging is for pre-operative localisation prior to surgical intervention. The advent of nuclear medicine and combination scans has had a massive impact on allowing minimal access surgery for parathyroid disease. It has allowed focused, more limited dissection and is associated with reduced hospital costs and a swifter return to work. It has also allowed for the easier identification of ectopic parathyroid glands, which was previously problematic. For rarer conditions, such as carcinomas or cysts, a range of adjunct investigations is now available. However, there is yet no completely foolproof test, and for this reason further trials and studies are mandatory.

References

[1] Kirkby-Bott J, El-Khatib Z, Soudan B, Caiazzo R, Arnalsteen L, Carnaille B. 25 hydroxy vitamin D deficiency causes parathyroid incidentalomas. *Langenbeck Arch. Surg.* 2010; 395; 919-924.

[2] Carnaille BM, Pattou FN, Oudar C, Lecomte-Houcke MC, Rocha JE, Proye CA. Parathyroid incidentalomas in normocalcemic patients during thyroid surgery. *World J. Surg.* 1996; 20:830-834.

[3] Wang, CA. The anatomic basis of parathytroid surgery. *Ann. Surg.* 1976; 183:271-275.

[4] Akerstrom G, Malmaeus J, Bergstrom R. Surgical anatomy of human parathyroid glands. *Surgery* 1984; 95:14-21.

[5] Fakhran S, Branstetter BF, Pryma DA. Parathyroid Imaging. *Neuroimag. Clin. N. Am.* 2008; 18:537-549.

[6] Johnson NA, Tublin ME, Ogilvie JB. Parathyroid Imaging: Technique and Role in the Preoperative Evaluation of Primary Hyperparathyroidism. *Am. J. Roentgenol.* 2007; 188: 1706-1715.

[7] Reeder SB, Desser TS, Weigel RJ, Jeffrey RB. Sonography in primary hyperparathyroidism: review with emphasis on scanning technique. *J. Ultrasound Med.* 2002; 21:539-552.

[8] Wolf RJ, Cronan JJ, Monchik JM. Color Doppler sonography: an adjunctive technique in assessment of parathyroid adenomas. *J. Ultrasound. Med.* 1994; 13:303-308.

[9] Mollerup CL, Bollerslev J, Blicherta-Toft M. Primary hyperparathyroidism: incidence and clinical and biochemical characteristics – a demographic study. *Eur J. Surg.* 1994; 160:485-489.

[10] Barraclough BM, Barraclough BH. Ultrasound of the thyroid and parathyroid glands. *World J. Surg.* 2000; 24(2):158–165.

[11] Kamaya A, Quon A, Jeffrey RB. Sonography of the abnormal parathyroid gland. *Ultrasound Q* 2006; 22(4):253–262.

[12] DeFeo ML, Colagrande S, Biagini C, *et al.* Parathyroid glands: combination of (99m)Tc MIBI scintigraphy and US for demonstration of parathyroid glands and nodules. *Radiology* 2000; 214(2):393–402.

[13] Kirkby-Bott J, Carnaille B. Experience of the reliability of intra-operative sampling of tissue PTH in parathyroid surgery (letter to the editor). *World J. Surg.* 2010; 34:2254.

[14] Horanyi J, Duffek L, Szla ́vik R *et al.* Intraoperative determination of PTH concentrations in fine needle tissue aspirates to identify parathyroid tissue during parathyroidectomy. *World J. Surg.* 2010; 34:538–543.

[15] Chan RK, Ibrahim SI, Pil P, *et al.* Validation of a method to replace frozen section during parathyroid exploration by using the rapid parathyroid hormone assay on parathyroid aspirates. *Arch. Surg.* 2005; 140:371–373.

[16] Lo CY, Chan WF, Leung P, *et al.* Applicability of tissue aspirate for quick parathyroid hormone assay to confirm parathyroid tissue identity during parathyroidectomy for primary hyper- parathyroidism. *Arch. Surg.* 2005; 140:146–149.

[17] Perrier ND, Ituarte P, Kikuchi S, *et al.* Intraoperative parathyroid aspiration and parathyroid hormone assay as an alternative to frozen section for tissue identification. *World J. Surg.* 2000; 24:1319–1322.

[18] Siperstein A, Berber E, Macket R, Alghoul M, Wagner K, Milas M. Prospective evaluation of sestamibi scan, ultrasonography and rapid PTH to predict the success of limited exploration for sporadic primary hyperparathyroidism. *Surgery* 2004; 136:872-880.

[19] Haber RS, Kim CK, Inabnet WB. Ultrasonography for preoperative localization of enlarged parathyroid glands in primary hyperparathyroidism: comparison with (99m) technetium sestamibi scintigraphy. *Clin. Endocrinol.* 2002; 57:241-249.

[20] Uruno T, Kebebew E. How to localize parathyroid tumors in primary hyperparathyroidism? *J. Endocrinol. Invest.* 2006; 29(9):840–847.

[21] Cercueil JP, Jacob D, Verges B, Holtzmann P, Lerais JM, Krause D. Percutaneous ethanol injection into parathyroid adenomas: mid- and long-term results. *Eur. Radiol.* 1998; 8:1565-1569.

[22] Nguyen BD. Parathyroid imaging with Tc-99m sestami bi planar and SPECT scintigraphy. *Radiographics* 1999;19(3):601–614.

[23] Lavely WC, Goetze S, Friedman KP, *et al.* Comparison of SPECT/CT, SPECT, and planar imaging with single- and dual-phase (99m)Tc-sestamibi parathyroid scintigraphy. *J. Nucl. Med.* 2007;48(7):1084–1089.

[24] Ruda JM, Hollenbeak CS, Stack BC Jr. A systematic review of the diagnosis and treatment of primary hyperparathyroidism from 1995 to 2003. *Otolaryngol. Head Neck Surg.* 2005; 132:359-372.

[25] Civelek AC, Ozalp E, Donovan P, Udelsman R. Prospective evaluation of delayed technetium-99m sestamibi SPECT scintigraphy for preoperative localization of primary hyperparathyroidism. *Surgery* 2002; 131:149-157.

[26] Vattimo A, Bertelli P, Cintorino M, *et al.* Identification of Hurthle cell tumor by single-injection, double phase scintigraphy with technetium-99m-sestamibi. *J. Nucl. Med.* 1995;36(5):778–782.

[27] Kandil E, Tufaro AP, Carson KA, Lin F, Somervel H, Farrag T, Dackiw A, Zeiger M, Tufano RP. Correlation of Plasma 25-Hydroxyvitamin D LevelsWith Severity of Primary Hyperparathyroidism and Likelihood of Parathyroid Adenoma Localization on Sestamibi Scan. *Arch. Otolaryngol. Head Neck Surg.* 2008; 134(10): 1073-1075.

[28] Kirkby-Bott J, Skandarajah A, Markogiannakis H, Cowan M, Fleming B, Palazzo F. Pre-operative vitamin D deficiency predicts post-operative hypocalcaemia after total thyroidectomy. *World J. Surg.* 2011; 35:324–330.

[29] Otto D, Boerner AR, Hofmann M, *et al.* Preoperative localisation of hyperfunctional parathyroid tissue with C-11methionine PET. *Eur. J. Nucl. Med. Mol. Imaging.* 2004; 31:1405-1412.

[30] Hellman P, Ahlstrom H, Bergstrom M, *et al.* Positron emission tomography with C-11 methionine in hyperparathyroidism. *Surgery* 1994; 116:974-981.

[31] Lumachi F, Zucchetta P, Marzola MC, *et al.* Advantages of combined technetium-99m-sestamibi scintigraphy and high-resolution ultrasonography in parathyroid localization: comparative study in 91 patients with primary hyperparathyroidism. *Eur. J. Endocrinol.* 2000; 143: 755-760.

[32] Öksüz M.Ö, Dittmann H, Wicke C, Müssig K, Bares R, Pfannenberg C, Eschmann S.M. Accuracy of parathyroid imaging: a comparison of planar scintigraphy, SPECT, SPECT-CT and C-11 methionine PET for the detection of parathyroid adenomas and glandular hyperplasia. *Diagn. Interv. Radiol.* DOI 10.4261/1305-3825.DIR.3486-10.1.

[33] Solorzano CC, carneiro-Pla DM, Irvin GL 3rd. Surgeon-performed ultrasonography as the initial and only localizing study in sporadic and primary hyperparathyroidism. *J. Am. Coll. Surg.* 2006; 202:18-24.

[34] Rodgers SE, Hunter GJ, Hamberg LM, *et al.* Improved preoperative planning for directed parathyroidectomy with 4-dimensional computed tomography. *Surgery* 2006; 140(6):932–940.

[35] Gotway MB, Higgins CB. MR imaging of the thyroid and parathyroid glands. *Magn. Reson. Imaging Clin. N. Am.* 2000; 8:163-182.

[36] Ernst O. Hyperparathyroïde: Applications du scanner et de l'IRM. *J. Radiol.* 2009;90:409-12.

[37] Clark P, Wooldridge T, Kleinpeter K, *et al.* Providing optimal preoperative localization for recurrent parathyroid carcinoma: a combined parathyroid scintigraphy and computed tomography approach. *Clin. Nucl. Med.* 2004; 29(11):681–684.

[38] Gotway MB, Reddy GP, Webb WR, Morita ET, Clark OH, Higgins CB. Comparison between MR imaging and 99mTc MIBI scintigraphy in the evaluation of recurrent or persistent hyperparathyroidism. *Radiology* 2001; 218:783-790.

[39] Lopez Hanninen E, Vogl TJ, Steinmuller T, *et al.* Preoperative contrast-enhanced MRI of the parathyroid glands in hyperparathyroidism. *Invest. Radiol.* 2000; 35(7):426–430.

[40] Lee VS, Spritzer CE. MR imaging of abnormal parathyroid glands. *Am. J. Roentgenol.* 1998;170(4): 1097–1103.

Part 2:
Parathyroid Function

In: Parathyroid: Anatomy, Functions and Disorders
Editor: James Kirkby-Bott
ISBN: 978-1-62100-765-4

Chapter III

Parathyroid Gland and Calcium Physiology

Rajeev Raghavan and Bushra Ahmad
Spire Briston Hospital, United Kingdom

Abstract

The parathyroid glands located in the neck, secrete parathyroid hormone (PTH) which is a key player in calcium homeostasis and bone health. The regulation of calcium homeostasis involves the interactions of PTH, Vitamin-D, calcitonin, and serum calcium with the latter acting via the calcium sensing receptor (CaSR).

In this chapter the histology of the parathyroid glands, structure of PTH, challenges in biochemical measurement of PTH, the structure and role of the calcium sensing receptor (CaSR), and the functional mutations in the CaSR contributing to disease models are explored. The role of Calcitonin in calcium metabolism and regulation of PTH secretion and action is reviewed.

Parathyroid related protein structure, secretion and its place in the diagnostic pathway for hypercalcaemia are discussed. Finally the mechanisms underlying hypocalcaemia and hypoparathyroidism and the clinical picture, management and monitoring is outlined.

Abbreviations

PTH = parathyroid Hormone;
1,25-D = active form of vitamin-D;
CaSR = Calcium sensing receptor;
GI = gastrointestinal;
CKD = chronic kidney disease;
PHP = pseudohypoparathyroidism;
VDR = Vitamin-D receptor;
VDRE = vitamin D response element

Introduction

The parathyroids derive their name from their close proximity to the thyroid gland and were first recognised by Ivor Sandstrom, a Swedish medical student, in 1880. In 1891, Eugene Emile Gley demonstrated the importance of parathyroid glands to calcium homeostasis by demonstrating tetany in laboratory animals that had undergone a total parathyroidectomy [1]. This was further corroborated by important histopathological work conducted by Jacob Erdheim demonstrating parathyroid tissue in specimens from thyroidectomised patients who had developed hypocalcaemia. Prior to this, symptoms arising from hypocalcaemia had been attributed to the thyroid gland [1]. Calcium is the fifth most abundant mineral in the human body and the only source of calcium is through the diet. Most of the total body store of calcium is found in the skeleton where it serves to strengthen the bone by forming hydroxyapatite in conjunction with phosphate. Therefore skeletal bone serves as a reservoir for calcium and phosphate allowing these minerals to flux into the circulation in a dynamic fashion.

The three calciotropic hormones, parathyroid hormone (PTH), calcitonin (CT), and vitamin D (particularly the active form 1,25-dihydroxyvitamin D [1,25-D]), through their actions and interactions on bone, kidney and the gastrointestinal (GI) tract, act to maintain both serum and extracellular fluid calcium within the normal range. Such precise regulation of serum calcium is essential for many calcium-requiring physiological functions such as neural transmission and muscle contraction. In addition, serum calcium plays an important role in self-regulation via regulating concentrations of the calciotropic hormones to maintain both calcium homeostasis and the homeostasis of allied micronutrients, chiefly magnesium and phosphate. This is achieved by an appropriate counterbalancing change in PTH secretion from the parathyroid, calcitonin from C-cells of the thyroid, and in vitamin-D levels. Such a response is dependent on the capacity of the bone to act as a dynamic pool for calcium, magnesium, and phosphate from which blood levels can be regulated. In the normal physiological state hypocalcaemia leads to an increase in serum PTH and 1,25-D and a decrease in serum calcitonin. The result of this process is an increase in GI absorption of calcium, increase in bone resorption, and decrease in renal calcium excretion. These alterations act to increase the serum calcium towards normal. Conversely in hypercalcaemia both serum PTH and 1,25-D are suppressed and serum calcitonin levels increase. This leads to a reduction in GI absorption of calcium, decrease in bone resorption, and an increase in renal calcium excretion all combining to restore serum calcium back to normal.

Table 1. Hormones involved in bone metabolism

Bone metabolism	Stimulated	Inhibited
Bone Formation	Vitamin D and analogues Growth Hormone Androgens Insulin PTH at low dose	Glucocorticoids
Bone Resorption	Parathormone (PTH) PTH related peptide Glucocorticoids Thyroid hormones Hypervitaminosis D	Calcitonin Oestrogens

In addition to these three calciotropic hormones, other hormones (such as insulin, growth hormone, thyroid hormone, and the gonadal and adrenal steroids [Table 1]), cytokines, and growth factors play an important role in calcium metabolism.

Calcium Homeostasis

Calcium Physiology

Calcium is a ubiquitous molecule that has wide ranging actions in a number of tissues. Calcium homeostasis in blood is maintained by calcium uptake from the gastrointestinal (GI) tract, calcium excretion via the kidneys, and exchange with the body's main calcium store, bone. There is a ready flux of calcium, magnesium, and phosphorus between the blood and the cells regulated by these three organ systems (GI tract, kidney, and bone) [2, 3] and governed by the three main calciotropic hormones, along with other influences. Blood ionised calcium levels and thereby intracellular calcium levels are maintained within a narrow range that is vital to the maintenance of all the functions for which calcium is required. Since the skeleton has an integral role in calcium metabolism, the regulation of calcium can be understood through an understanding of skeletal homeostasis.

Average dietary intake of calcium is around 1g/day, although there is wide variability. There is net absorption across the gut wall of approximately 50% of ingested calcium. The proximal small intestine (duodenum and jejunum) is a major site for calcium absorption which explains the significant calcium deficit that occurs in disorders of the small intestine such as coeliac disease. Calcium absorption occurs by passive diffusion, ion exchange, and active transport-mediated by calcium binding proteins (also called calbindins).

The skeleton holds 99% of the body's calcium stores. Most of the remainder is in the circulation and just over 50% of this is found free in the form of ionised calcium [4], with the rest mainly being bound to blood proteins or forming complexes with other compounds (Figure-1). It is ionised calcium that is active although most assays in practice only estimate the total calcium which is then "corrected" for the serum albumin content. Roughly 10g/day is filtered by the kidneys but a majority of this is reabsorbed with approximately 1% being found in the urine.

Urinary calcium (UCa) is excreted in proportion to serum calcium (PCa) until a certain serum calcium threshold is reached, which then results in a steep rise in calcium excretion. Representation of this interaction between serum and urine calcium forms a steep curve in the normal physiological state. The steepness of the curve is due to the nature of the interaction between extracellular calcium and the CaSR [5].

It is shifted to the left in the absence of calciotropic factors such as PTH and 1,25-D and remains completely flat in conditions such as familial hypocalciuric hypercalcaemia.

Bone turnover is mediated via osteoclasts and osteoblasts which in turn are controlled via their cell surface receptors by the three calciotropic hormones (PTH, vitamin D, and calcitonin) and other chemicals such as steroids and growth hormone (GH). The major actions of the three main hormones are discussed through the course of this chapter.

Osteoclasts are responsible chiefly for bone resorption and therefore calcium exit from bone and osteoblasts form the bone matrix and therefore take up calcium from the blood.

However, the interactions between the various cells in the skeleton are complex given the variation in bone turnover between different sites in the body. All the same, conditions such as hyperparathyroidism cause increase in movement of calcium from bone into the blood (increased osteoclastic activity) and by extension into urine and hypoparathyroidism leads to increased renal excretion of calcium with less calcium flux into the blood, thus contributing to the ensuing hypocalcaemia.

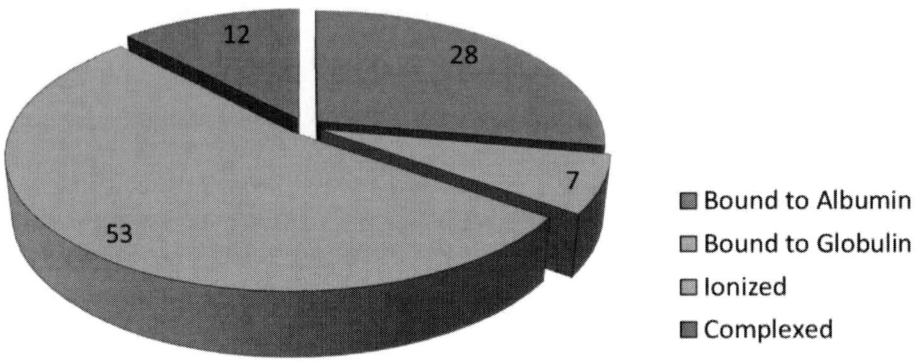

Figure 3.1. Composition of serum calcium in the range of 2.3-2.7 mmol/l.

The Calcium Sensing Receptor (CaSR)

In the mid-1990s scientists working at the Harvard Medical School described the calcium sensing receptor which belongs to the G-protein receptor superfamily. [6] Such G-protein receptors characteristically have seven trans-membrane domains and are also referred to as heptahelical or serpentine receptors [7]. They bind a variety of ligands across the animal kingdom including pheromones, hormones, and neurotransmitters [8]. Apart from the parathyroid glands, the CaSR can be found in the C-cells of the thyroid, kidneys, brain, and several other tissues [7] suggesting that it may play a role in local calcium regulation independent of calciotropic factors and that calcium may have a direct "hormone" like effect on these tissues. The CaSR also regulates the response of thyroid C cells to changes in serum calcium concentration with appropriate secretion of calcitonin. In addition the CaSR is found in the distal nephron of the kidney where calcium excretion is regulated, in the placenta where foetal-maternal calcium fluxes occur, and in bone where its function is unclear.

Activation of the CaSR by calcium causes two major signal transduction effects involving activation of phospholipase C with subsequent activation of second messengers and inhibition of adenylate cyclase and suppression of intracellular concentration of cyclic AMP. These pathways have been implicated in the regulation of PTH and Calcitonin secretion. Thus an increase in serum calcium causes activation of the CaSR to reduce PTH secretion and thereby reduce calcium levels. Compounds have been identified that act selectively on the CaSR and may be useful treatment options for increased PTH secretion that occurs in primary and in particular secondary hyperparathyroidism. One of these cinacalcet is now licensed for treatment of secondary hyperparathyroidism for patients with chronic kidney disease [9].

Parathyroid Hormone Biology

Brief histology of Parathyroid Glands

Parathyroid hormone is secreted by two pairs of parathyroid glands located near the posterior aspect of the thyroid gland in the neck. Ectopic glands may be found anywhere along the line of descent of the branchial pouches. Parathyroid glands are divided into lobules with thin partitions in between. The tissue is mainly composed of stroma with variable (mean 17%, can be as much as 30%) fat content which mirrors visceral fat content. [10] Scattered within this stroma are two main cells types; chief cells (chief cells with abundant clear cytoplasm are called clear cells) and oxyphil cells. Chief cells exhibit maximum sensitivity to changes in ionised calcium and contain dense secretory granules packed with fully assembled PTH. [10] Oxyphil cells do not contain secretory granules and have no known function. The parathyroid gland cells have receptors for calcium (CaSR), Vitamin-D (vitamin-D receptor or VD-R), and the more recently elucidated fibroblast growth factor (FGF receptor) [11] all of which play a part in the responses of the gland in health and disease.

PTH Secretion and Regulation

PTH is an 84 amino acid peptide which is initially produced as a pre-pro-hormone of 115 amino acids in the chief cells of the parathyroid glands. This pre-pro hormone undergoes splicing of a 25 amino acid fragment and a 6 amino acid fragment leading to the formation of the active parathyroid hormone [12]. This hormone is packaged into secretory granules which are near the surface of the chief cells. The amino terminus of PTH and the associated amino acids numbered 1 to 34 are thought to be the active end of the molecule and this fragment in the circulation is called 1-34 PTH. The major regulatory signal for PTH secretion is serum calcium [5]. PTH levels can change very rapidly in the circulation in response to changes in serum calcium via the CaSR with CaSR activation inversely affecting PTH secretion. The interaction between calcium and PTH levels is maximal in the middle of the normal range for both substances which can be represented by a sigmoidal curve (see figure-2) [13, 14]. Even a small increase in serum ionized calcium inhibits PTH secretion by increasing intracellular calcium in the chief cells through the release of calcium from intracellular stores and the influx of extracellular calcium through cell membranes and channels. This mechanism differs from most cells where an increase in intracellular calcium (acting as a second messenger) would cause an increase in the normal output of the cells. Serum calcium inversely regulates transcription of the PTH gene, and PTH gene transcription is also inhibited by increased levels of 1,25-dihydroxyvitamin D (1,25-D).

Intracellular magnesium in the parathyroid cells behaves in the same way as calcium, with hypermagnesaemia inhibiting PTH secretion and hypomagnesaemia stimulating PTH secretion. However, prolonged depletion of magnesium will eventually inhibit PTH biosynthesis and secretion, and also the function of many cells. Furthermore hypomagnesaemia attenuates the biological effect of PTH by interfering with its signal transduction.

In hypocalcaemia (especially if chronic) serum calcium levels and its interactions with the CaSR will lead to proliferation of parathyroid cells and hence hyperplasia and conversely hypercalcaemia will inhibit parathyroid cell proliferation. In chronic kidney disease (CKD) upregulation of PTH secretion occurs which aims to maintain activity of 1-α hydroxylase enzyme in the kidney which is important for the conversion of 25-OH vitamin D to active vitamin-D. Moreover chronic kidney disease is associated with downregulation in expression of VDRs [15] and there is evidence that 1,25-D helps with autoregulation by increasing VDR synthesis [16]. Furthermore the secondary hyperparathyroidism that occurs in a proportion of uraemic patients may over time become unresponsive to vitamin-D metabolites due to nodular hyperplasia and monoclonal change in the parathyroid glands [15].

Current practice of proactively managing secondary hyperparathyroidism with 1-α calcidol mitigates this problem and the subsequent severe metabolic bone disease that can be seen with chronic kidney disease.

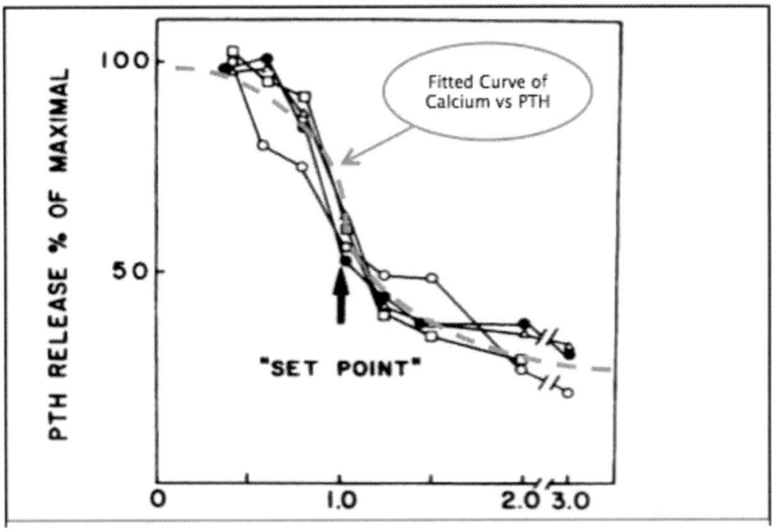

Figure 3.2. Graphical representation of the circulating PTH response to serum ionised calcium. Adapted with permission from: Brown E.M, MacLeod R.J Physiol Rev 2001;81:239-297.

Parathyroid Hormone Metabolism

Following secretion from the parathyroid glands, PTH is cleared within minutes from the circulation. The hormone is metabolized to amino-terminal (N-terminal) and carboxyl-terminal (C-terminal) fragments primarily in the liver but also in the kidney, and perhaps in the parathyroid gland and blood. The amino terminus end of PTH (1-34 PTH) has until recently been thought to exert all of the main biological actions of PTH.

The carboxyl terminal however, whilst having the potential to complicate assay results, may also have some biological effects which have been unclear but are now being recognised [17].

All of the by-products of PTH metabolism, in addition to the active form are detected to varying degrees by immunoassays. The intact PTH molecule (1-84) comprises 10-20% of all the circulating forms of PTH and the rest consists of a collection of various fragments including the N-terminal and C-terminal fragments and various mid-section fragments. Intact PTH and C-terminal fragments are cleared by glomerular filtration and hence accumulate in renal failure [18; 19]. It is suggested that a proportion of C-terminal fragments are also synthesised in the liver [20] and further contribute to circulating levels. Recent studies have shown that another fragment of PTH containing amino acids 7-84, may be secreted actively both by the normal and abnormal parathyroid gland.

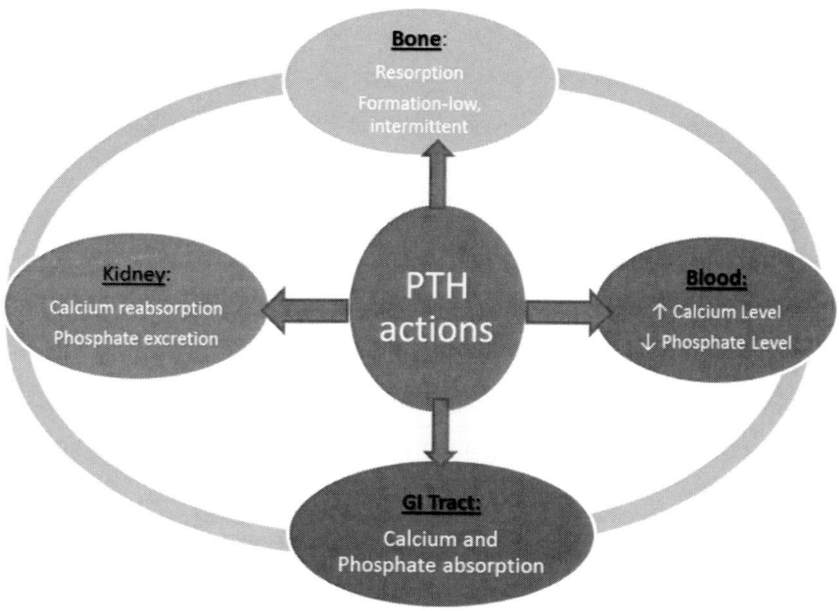

Figure 3.3. Actions of PTH schematically illustrated.

Conditions such as renal impairment can lead to an inflation of PTH assay results with relatively less PTH bioactivity and in clinical practice this along with assay cross-reactivity can cause difficulties with interpretation of PTH results. 2nd generation assays are designed to detect intact PTH (PTH 1-84) and were toted as more accurate compared to 1st generation PTH assays which tended to detect PTH fragments thus overestimating PTH levels. However in recent years it has been demonstrated that the 2nd generation assays also have a tendency to detect the 7-84 fragment of PTH (without the active amino terminus) especially in uraemic patients [21] and therefore leading to similar errors as the 1st generation assays. To counter this so called "bio-active" PTH assays have been designed [22] but the accuracy of these assays in detection of bio-active PTH is yet to be determined in clinical practice [23].

Functions of Parathyroid Hormone

Hormonal function of PTH (Figure-3) in bone is mediated through the PTH receptor located mainly on the osteoblast. When consistently elevated, PTH seems to predominantly influence osteoclastic activity leading to bone resorption. Conversely, intermittent exposure of bone to low levels of PTH increases osteoblastic activity. Osteoclastic activity is mediated via the RANKL–OPG pathway [24]. PTH influences GI absorption of calcium and phosphate mostly indirectly via activating vitamin-D. In addition, it does have a weak direct effect on luminal calcium and phosphate absorption. PTH promotes hypophosphataemia, hypercalcaemia, and a mild hyperchloraemic metabolic alkalosis via its renal effects of promoting phosphate loss in the proximal tubule, calcium reabsorption in the distal convoluted tubule, inhibition of Na+/H+ antiporter activity, and bicarbonate loss in the urine. [25].

PTH Receptors

Until recently only one PTH receptor had been described. This receptor with a molecular weight of 80,000 belongs to the G protein receptor super family and is now called the Type-1 PTH receptor (PTH-1R). PTH related peptide (PTHrP) is a protein product of various tissues within the body and its molecular structure has much similarity to PTH but has a number of different actions. PTHrP and its clinical implications are discussed at the end of this chapter. The PTH-1R has affinity in equal measure for both the amino-terminal of PTH and its counterpart on the PTHrP [12]. This affinity is shared via the amino terminal of both peptides which has a 13 amino acid homology between the two molecules [26; 27]. With the binding of PTH/PTHrP to the PTH1R, there is activation of multiple downstream pathways via coupling to G-proteins. Some of these pathways are schematically represented in Figure-4. Both PTH and PTHrP via adenylate cyclase generate cyclic adenosine monophosphate (cAMP) as a cellular second messenger which in turn activates protein kinase A (PKA) [27]. This then leads to phosphorylation of transcription factors. Activation of the phospholipase C effector system by PTH binding has the dual effect of increasing intracellular inositol triphosphate which in turn increases cytosolic calcium and of activating protein kinase C (PKC) via diacylglycerol [28]. There is some tissue specificity as to which pathway dominates. The Type-2 PTH receptor (PTH-2R) has no role in calcium and mineral metabolism and is PTH specific (i.e. has no affinity for PTHrP).

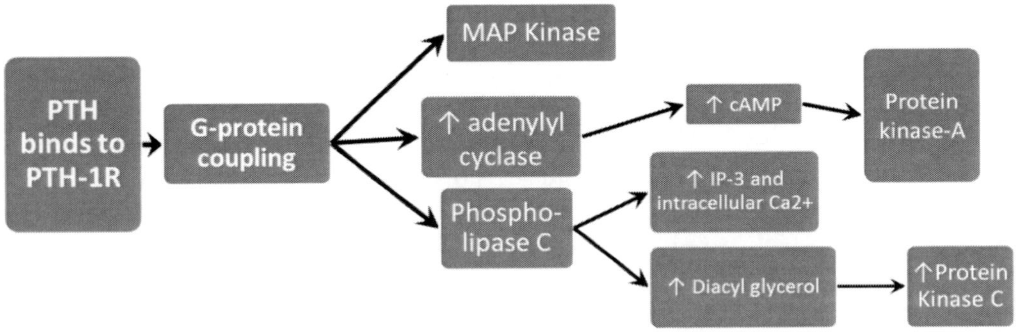

Figure 3.4. Intracellular pathways for PTH action via the PTH-1 receptor.

Although the brain, pancreas, testes, and placenta are some of the tissues expressing the PTH-2R, it is unclear if PTH exerts any effects in-vivo via this receptor. The role of the PTH-2R has yet to be elucidated in humans [12].

Vitamin-D – Role in Calcium Metabolism

Vitamin-D and its analogues are steroid hormones called secosteroids due to the partial steroid ring within their structure. The main source of vitamin-D is derived by exposure to sunlight. A vitamin-D precursor in the skin called 7-dehydrocholesterol is converted by sunlight in the ultraviolet-B spectrum to vitamin-D3. Diet containing naturally available or supplemental vitamin-D2 (called ergocalciferol) or vitamin-D3 (called colecalciferol) is the other source of vitamin-D particularly in the Western World. Vitamin-D2 and vitamin-D3 are inactive forms of vitamin-D which, within the body, are activated by a two-step process in the liver and kidneys to active 1,25 dihydroxy vitamin-D (1,25-D also known as calcitriol) (see figure-5) [29]. PTH is required for the final activation step of vitamin-D in the kidneys. Vitamin-D maintains calcium and phosphate homeostasis by aiding absorption of both these molecules from the intestine and skeletal stores (particularly in hypocalcaemia) and enabling reabsorption of calcium and phosphate excreted in the kidneys.

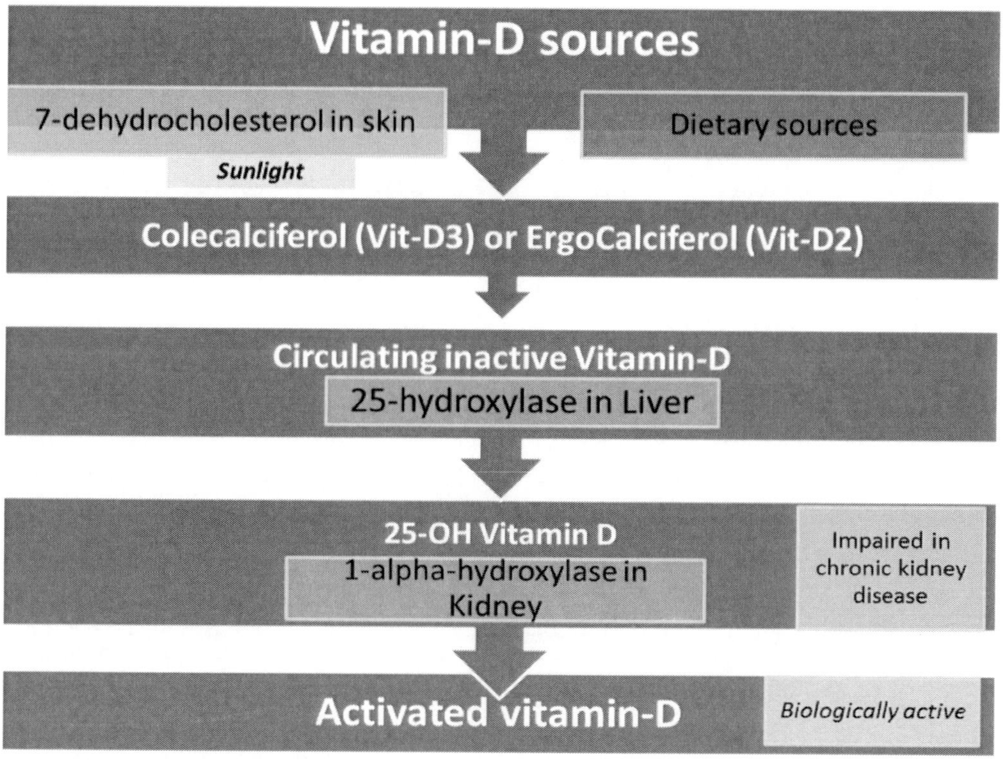

Figure 3.5. Sources of vitamin-D and pathway for activation of vitamin-D.

Binding of vitamin-D to the vitamin-D receptor (VDR) causes activation of transcriptional factors called vitamin-D response elements or VDREs which lead to the actions of vitamin-D. 1,25-D and its metabolites have multiple effects on intracellular pathways implicated in bone health, cardiovascular health, and cell proliferation [29].

Calcitonin and its Role in Calcium Metabolism

Calcitonin (CT), a product of the thyroid parafollicular or C-cells, by lowering serum calcium calcitonin has the opposite effect to vitamin-D and PTH and thereby facilitates maintenance of calcium homeostasis. Calcium feedback to calcitonin action also occurs through the CaSR. Calcitonin action is mediated through the CT receptor rich osteoclast. The calcitonin receptor belongs to the same family of serpentine receptors as the PTH receptor and has several isoforms found in several tissue types [7]. The calcitonin gene also produces a smaller 37 amino acid polypeptide called calcitonin gene related product (CGRP) in neural tissues [30] which has only weak affinity to the CT receptors in the skeleton. Effects of Calcitonin on mineral metabolism can be broken down into its effects on bone, kidneys, GI tract, and blood. In bone calcitonin inhibits osteoclastic activity reducing bone resorption and probably also actively promotes bone formation [31]. Calcitonin leads to a reduction in phosphate reabsorption in the kidneys and promotes calcium loss in the urine [32]. In the GI tract calcitonin has an inhibitory effect on calcium and phosphorus absorption. All of these actions serve to decrease serum calcium and phosphorus [33]. Calcitonin in addition, serves as an important tumour marker in medullary thyroid cancer (MTC) and neuroendocrine tumours.

Disturbance in Calcium Homeostasis – Hypocalcaemia

Hypocalcaemia is defined as serum calcium less than 2.20 mmol/L (corrected for serum albumin) or ionised calcium of 0.97mmol/L [4]. In the normal physiological state Vitamin-D and PTH work together, to maintain serum calcium in the normal range.

Hypocalcaemia, therefore results from a disturbance in the function of these hormones. Causes for hypocalcaemia include hypoparathyroidism (either a direct deficit of PTH or lack of action at the target organ level), hypovitaminosis-D (either due to a direct deficit or due to a lack of action), hyperphosphataemia, drug induced hypocalcaemia, and calcium precipitation. A list of causes of hypocalcaemia can be found in Table-2. Since calcium is vital for intracellular activities and is a key part of synaptic transmission [34], the main symptoms of hypocalcaemia relate to neuromuscular instability. Thus muscular spasms, paraesthesia, and tetany (involuntary tonic muscular contractions) can subsequently lead to seizures and organic brain disease.

Carpo-pedal spasm is a manifestation of tetany characterised by flexion of the carpo-metacarpal joints, extension of the interphalangeal joints, adduction of the thumb and flexion of the wrist causing a painful posture. This is usually a manifestation of severe hypocalcaemia and sometimes if not overtly present can be elicited by certain stimuli such as pressure over the arm from inflation of a blood pressure cuff (Trosseau's sign) or stimulation of the facial nerve by tapping on the cheek just below the zygomatic bone about $3/4^{th}$ inch in front of the earlobe (Chvostek's sign). Chvostek's sign is caused by contraction of the facial musculature to varying degrees in response to external stimulus, indicating mild to moderate neuromuscular instability. Both Trosseau's and Chvostek's signs can sometimes be seen in individuals with normocalcaemia and therefore are not entirely specific to hypocalcaemia.

Table 2. Causes of Hypocalcaemia classified based on underlying aetiology

PTH	**Hypoparathyroidism** • Surgical • Idiopathic • Neonatal • Familial • Autoimmune • Deposition of metals (iron, copper, aluminum) • Postradiation • Infiltrative • Functional (in hypomagnesaemia)	**Resistance to PTH action** • Pseudohypoparathyroidism • Renal insufficiency • Medications that block osteoclastic bone resorption Bisphosphonates (especially IV) Calcitonin Plicamycin
Vitamin-D	**Failure of 1, 25 Dihydroxy Vitamin-D synthesis** – Vitamin D deficiency – Hereditary vitamin D-dependent rickets-type 1 (deficiency of renal 1α-hydroxylase)	**Target organ resistance** – Hereditary vitamin D-dependent rickets-type 2 (defective Vitamin-D receptor)
Calcium deposition or complex formation	**Acute hyperphosphatemia** • Crush injury with myonecrosis • Rapid tumor lysis • Parenteral phosphate administration • Excessive enteral phosphate Phosphate-containing antacids, Phosphate-containing enemas	**Acute pancreatitis** **Citrated blood transfusion** **Rapid, excessive skeletal mineralization** • Hungry bones syndrome • Osteoblastic metastasis • Vitamin D therapy for vitamin D deficiency

Symptoms and signs may also arise due to lack of calcium in the ectodermal tissues and include dry skin, brittle nails, alopecia, enamel hypoplasia, poor dentition, and increased dental caries. Calcium is deposited in tissues particularly when there is attendant hyperphosphataemia as in hypoparathyroidism or PTH resistance leading to cataracts and neurological problems (basal ganglia calcification causing extra-pyramidal symptoms). Cardiac effects of hypocalcaemia include rhythm disturbances, cardiomyopathy, and heart failure. Acute and severe hypocalcaemia can cause organic brain syndrome and seizures which may be difficult to treat without normalising the serum calcium. Chronic hypocalcaemia in children can cause mental retardation. Hypocalcaemia from vitamin-D deficiency is accompanied by hypophosphataemia and affects the skeleton with growth plate disorders in children (rickets) and inadequate bone mineralisation in adults (osteomalacia) [35]. It is important to be aware that chronic hypocalcaemia may be asymptomatic or only cause mild symptoms.

Surgical Causes of Hypoparathyroidism

A deficiency of PTH most commonly occurs as a result of surgical disruption of the parathyroid glands due to parathyroidectomy or as bystander damage in thyroid or head and neck surgery. Incidence of transient hypocalcaemia can be as high as 23% following neck surgery and factors such as radiotherapy can exacerbate parathyroid damage. However permanent hypoparathyroidism was only seen in 0.9% of patients who underwent neck dissection as reported in one study [36], whereas surgery for hyperparathyroidism can cause a higher incidence of hypoparathyroidism.

Various studies have tried to elucidate predictors for post-operative and subsequent long term hypocalcaemia. These factors include the size of the goitre, need for extensive dissection, surgical expertise, loss of three parathyroid glands [37], post-operative calcium and post-operative PTH levels [38]. A high incidence of transient mild hypocalcaemia on the first post-operative day has been put down to haemodilution and transient injury to parathyroid glands. It is thought that the parathyroid remnant may have temporarily lost its blood supply which is then re-established. It has been suggested that a calcium level measured on the second post-operative day has better predictive value [38]. Some centres use parathyroid auto-transplantation in order to try and prevent hypoparathyroidism. Another strategy where neck dissection is anticipated is to treat with prophylactic calcium and vitamin-D supplements [39].While this strategy is safe and does not usually cause hypercalcaemia it is not universally applicable (e.g. patients with hyperparathyroidism awaiting surgery) and does increase the difficulty in monitoring post-operative biochemistry. As interest in day case parathyroid surgery is increasing one strategy that is being put forth is to put all patients on calcium and vitamin-D supplements post-operatively without prior demonstration of hypocalcaemia and then reassessing at a set time interval.

"Hungry bones" syndrome is a term used to describe significant hypocalcaemia following successful parathyroid surgery in subjects with severe hyperparathyroidism [40; 41]. It is a result of sudden avid uptake of calcium and phosphate by bone which has hitherto, under the influence of excess parathyroid hormone, been losing calcium. This is further discussed in the section on "Treatment of hypoparathyroid hypocalcaemia".

Non-Surgical Causes of Hypoparathyroidism

The causes of non-surgical hypoparathyroidism can be classified into autoimmune, genetic, or other metabolic insults causing hypoparathyroidism (e.g. hypomagnesaemia) [42] (see Table-2). Hypoparathyroidism associated with polyglandular syndrome and idiopathic hypoparathyroidism have both been associated with circulatory antibodies [43] directed against the CaSR rather than directly against parathyroid hormone [44], leading to activation of the CaSR and thereby directly to hypocalcaemia. The parathyroid gland is the chief endocrine organ affected in polyglandular autoimmune syndrome type-1. Mutations in the transcription factor regulating immune and endocrine function called autoimmune regulator (AIRE) protein are thought to be implicated in this condition [45].

Functional Mutations in the CaSR Leading to Hypocalcaemia

A number of genetic and functional disorders of the CaSR have been described. Over 20 mutations have been identified in the CaSR gene which can lead to autosomal dominant hypoparathyroidism [46-49] causing varying degrees of hypocalcaemia.

Gain of function mutations of the CaSR lead to hypoparathyroidism and therefore hypocalcaemia. Such mutations lead to a putatively active receptor with an elevated sensitivity to serum calcium. The result of this is a reduction in PTH secretion at a lower set point for serum calcium, increase in urinary calcium excretion, decrease in serum calcium, and ultimately leads to hypercalciuric hypocalcaemia. [50].

Mutations that affect the CaSR in the kidney lead to calciuria at a lower threshold of serum calcium [51]. The implications include increased tendency to nephrolithiasis especially in patients with renal impairment who are being treated with activated vitamin-D.

Syndromic Causes of Hypoparathyroidism

Conditions causing congenital/inherited hypoparathyroidism include DiGeorge syndrome (hypoparathyroidism, immune dysfunction, cardiac defects, and facial dysmorphism) [52], HDR syndrome (Hypoparathyroidism, Deafness, and Renal problems) [53], mitochondrial disorders (e.g. Kearns-Sayers syndrome), microdeletion of 22q11 syndrome [54], and autosomal recessive polyglandular syndrome type-1 (mucocutaneous candidiasis, Addison's disease, and hypoparathyroidism).

Severe hypomagnesaemia can affect PTH release from the parathyroid and also blunt PTH action when faced with hypocalcaemia. Correction with magnesium supplementation reverses this problem.

Pseudohypoparathyroidism (PHP)

This term encompasses a broad set of conditions where idiopathic or inherited resistance to PTH action at the receptor level is present. Albright and his colleagues were the first in 1942 to describe Albright's hereditary osteodystrophy (AHO) [55] in a group of patients with skeletal deformities (typically short 4th metacarpal), round facies, short stature, subcutaneous calcification, and metabolic defects which were similar to those in patients with hypoparathyroidism but with high PTH levels suggesting PTH resistance. Further work in this area has identified subtypes of this disorder characterised by defects in the GNAS gene (which encodes the α-subunit of Gs-α an ubiquitous signalling protein involved in cellular actions of several hormones, neurotransmitters, and paracrine factors)[56; 57]. This disorder has varying phenotypic expression and metabolic manifestations.

PHP type-1a features both AHO and tissue resistance to PTH, PHP type-1b however has biochemical features akin to AHO but without the phenotype characteristics of AHO. Pseudopseudohypoparathyroidism (PPHP) is a variant of this condition where patients have the phenotypic features of AHO but with no PTH resistance. Hypocalcaemia and hyperphosphataemia are well known in PHP but it is important to note that many patients may have minimal or no clinical features. Neurological features may sometimes occur and hypocalcaemia may lead to epilepsy. Co-existence of other hormone resistance such as thyroid stimulating hormone (TSH resistance), growth hormone (GH) resistance can also be found [58].

Treatment of Hypoparathyroid Hypocalcaemia

The main goal of treatment is to keep calcium within the normal range while avoiding iatrogenic hypercalcaemia and other consequences arising from calciuria such as renal calculi and nephrocalcinosis both of which can lead to renal impairment and renal failure. Given the important role of vitamin-D in calcium metabolism and in the absorption of calcium from the gut it is imperative to measure vitamin-D levels and consider replacing vitamin-D either in the form of vitamin-D2 or vitamin-D3. In case of renal impairment there is deficit of the renal enzyme 1-alpha hydroxylase and therefore replacement strategies include the use of 1-alfacalcidol (1-alpha hydroxyl group has been incorporated) or Calcitriol (1,25-D). Calcium levels at the lower end of the normal range or just below the normal limit would be desirable provided the patient is asymptomatic as this will minimise urinary calcium efflux as the retention of calcium by PTH has been lost. Hypoparathyroidism due to parathyroidectomy or impaired PTH secretion or ineffective circulating PTH leads to impairment of vitamin-D activation in the kidney. In this situation large doses of calcium supplementation may be required to get an effective increase in serum calcium. Alternatively using an activated vitamin-D preparation such as calcitriol will enable correction of hypocalcaemia with minimal calcium supplementation. In severe hyperparathyroidism, parathyroidectomy can lead to profound uptake of calcium by the skeleton rapidly diminishing circulating calcium. When this is coupled with the relative lack of PTH insufficient mobilisation of the calcium stores in the skeleton can cause a state of severe hypocalcaemia called "hungry bone syndrome" [41]. This could occur even with PTH being in the normal range as the remaining parathyroid gland/s have been relatively suppressed by the adenomatous or hyperplastic gland (particularly with removal of a large parathyroid gland and/or high pre-operative PTH levels) [41] and therefore are unable to respond to this sudden metabolic shift. This situation is further worsened in the presence of profound vitamin-D deficiency [59] and therefore some people would advocate measuring and cautiously correcting vitamin-D deficiency pre-operatively (aiming for a level of vitamin-D 50ng/l), to minimise this possibility. Current evidence suggests that such vitamin-D repletion therapy is relatively safe provided close monitoring of calcium levels is undertaken [60]. Following parathyroidectomy severe hypocalcaemia may need treatment with intravenous calcium (e.g. Calcium Gluconate) as per local guidance, followed by calcium and vitamin-D tablets (e.g. Calcichew-D3 containing 1.2 gm elemental calcium and 400 iu of vitamin-D per tablet). If there is persistent hypoparathyroidism then institution of Calcitriol is suggested in place of vitamin-D2 or vitamin-D3. The aim is to increase Calcitriol until calcium levels are maintained with only dietary calcium intake. Close monitoring of calcium is essential to prevent iatrogenic hypercalcaemia. Recent studies have demonstrated that treatment with Teriparatide (a synthetic abbreviated 1-34 amino terminal version of PTH) [61] and intact PTH [62], can maintain serum calcium as effectively as conventional treatment with calcium and vitamin-D preparations while achieving lesser levels of calciuria. However, at the moment cost implications prohibit routine use of these agents in current clinical practice.

Hypercalcaemia, PTH, and PTHrP

Hypercalcaemia defined as a serum calcium 2.7mmol/L has a number of causes as outlined in Table-3. The chief cause of hypercalcaemia in a hospital population is malignancy [63]. Malignancy leads to raised calcium levels by several mechanisms such as skeletal lysis, direct infiltration of the skeleton, metastatic deposits of tumour cells, or by secretion of a "humoral" factor leading to bone resorption. The term "humoral" is in reference to a circulating factor responsible for the elevated calcium and it is likely that either a circulating hormone or a hormone produced locally is ultimately responsible for increased osteoclastic activity [64].

Table 3. Causes of Hypercalcaemia divided by primary aetiology

Aetiology	Neoplasia	Inflammatory	Pharmacological	Miscellanoeus
PTH related	Ectopic production from tumour-rare	-----------------	--------------------------	Tertiary hyperparathyroidism
PTH-rP related	• Lung, • Breast, • Ovarian, • Lymphoproliferative • Neuroendocrine	------------------	------------------------------	------------------------------
Other --Systemic --Skeletal --Renal --Endocrine	• Metastases to bone, • Multiple Myeloma • Phaeochromocytoma	Sarcoid, Histiocytosis-X	• Thiazide diuretics • Hypervitaminosis-D • Hypervitaminosis-A • Theophylline toxicity • Lithium • Milk-Alkali Syndrome • Iatrogenic excess	• Immobility • Familial hypocalciuric hypercalcaemia • Hypophosphatasia • Advanced Chronic Liver disease • Hyperthyroidism • Adrenal insufficiency

Mutations in the CaSR Leading to Hypercalcaemia

Inactivating defects (loss of function mutations) of the CaSR lead to reduced sensitivity of the CaSR to serum calcium. This occurs in familial hypocalciuric hypercalcaemia which is a disorder characterised by decreased renal calcium excretion, normal to mildly elevated blood calcium levels, and a higher set point for inhibition of parathyroid hormone secretion via the CaSR [65]. The disorder results from a number of different mutations identified in different kindreds leading to different calcium sensing thresholds.

Ectopic PTH and PTHrP

In the 1960's and 1970's there were a number of cases of malignancy where "ectopic" production of PTH was reported as the cause of hypercalcaemia based on positive immunoreactivity to the PTH assays that were being used at the time. As discussed earlier in this chapter 1-34 PTH is responsible for the main biological effects of PTH. Therefore PTH fragments or circulating molecules which have the amino-terminus have shown cross-reactivity to previous assay platforms. Subsequent work has demonstrated that true "ectopic PTH" production is very rare and several cases of hypercalcaemia that had been previously attributed to this condition were most likely as a result of another protein which bore some resemblance to PTH and interacted with the PTH receptor, but had a very different structure [66]. In the 1980's the advent of highly specific and sensitive assays for PTH led to the discovery that sera from cancer patients who had hypercalcaemia due to suspected ectopic PTH production did not show any PTH immunoreactivity [66]. Further series of experiments demonstrated that a protein with PTH-like activity in such samples was not neutralised by antisera specific to human PTH. Purification of this protein from a human lung cancer cell line revealed a 17-18 kDa sized molecule which while being different in its overall structure from PTH shared homology of the amino terminus (8 out of 13 amino acids). This protein was given the term PTH-related protein or peptide (PTHrP).

True ectopic PTH secretion has been documented in very rare cases and mainly tends to result from small cell tumours. In one such case reported in 2005, a patient with small cell carcinoma of the ovary with hypercalcaemia had low levels of PTHrP and elevated levels of intact immunoactive PTH and the tumour cells in this case expressed PTH mRNA which was in keeping with PTH secreting ability [67]. There are other reports of such ectopic secretion from other tumour types such as pancreatic neuroendocrine tumours [64] and squamous cell tumours of the lung. In all these rare occurences, since the elucidation of PTHrP, the burden of proof for true ectopic PTH secretion has rested on demonstrating low PTHrP levels, normal parathyroid glands, and genetic evidence from the tumour cells of PTH production capabilities. This remains a rare clinical entity [64; 68].

References

[1] Potts JT. Parathyroid hormone past and present. *J. Endocrinol.* 2005, 187: 311-325.

[2] Bruder JM, Guise TA, and Mundy GR: Mineral Metabolism. In: Endocrinology and Metabolism, Fourth Edition, P. Felig and LA Frohman (eds.); Chapter 22, pp.1079-1159, 2001.

[3] Favus MJ: Intestinal Absorption of Calcium, Magnesium, and Phosphorus. In: Disorder of Bone and Mineral Metabolism, FL Coe and MJ Favus (eds.); Chapter 3, pp. 57-82, 1992.

[4] Conceicao SC, Weightman D, Smith PA, Luno J, Ward MK, Kerr DN. Serum ionised calcium concentration: measurement versus calculation. *Br. Med. J.* 1978 Apr 29;1(6120):1103-5.

[5] Brown EM, Hebert SC. Calcium receptor regulated parathyroid and renal function. *Bone* 20:303-309, 1997.

[6] Brown EM, Gamba G, Riccardi D, Lombardi M, Butters R, Kifor O, Sun A, Hediger MA, Lytton J, Hebert SC. Cloning and characterization of an extracellular Ca(2+)-sensing receptor from bovine parathyroid. *Nature*. 1993 Dec 9;366(6455):575-80.

[7] Brown EM, Segre GV, and Goldring SR: Serpentine receptors for parathyroid hormone, calcitonin and extracellular calcium ions. *Baillieres Clin. Endocrinol Metab. 10*:123-161, 1996.

[8] King N, Hittinger CT, Carroll SB. "Evolution of key cell signalling and adhesion protein families predates animal origins". *Science* 301 (5631): 361–3, 2003.

[9] Block GA, Martin KJ, de Francisco AL, Turner SA, Avram MM, Suranyi MG, Hercz G, Cunningham J, Abu-Alfa AK, Messa P, Coyne DW, Locatelli F, Cohen RM, Evanepoel P, Moe SM, Fournier A, Braun J, McCary LC, Zani VJ, Olson KA, Drüeke TB, and Goodman WG. Cinacalcet for secondary hyperparathyroidism in patients receiving hemodialysis, *N. Engl. J. Med.* 350: 1516-1525, 2004.

[10] Dufour DR, Wilkerson SY. The normal parathyroid revisited: percentage of stromal fat. *Hum. Pathol.* 1982 Aug;13(8):717-21.

[11] Ben-Dov IZ, Galitzer H, Lavi-Moshayoff V, Goetz R, Kuro OM, Mohammadi M, Sirkis R, Naveh-Many T, and Silver J: The parathyroid is a target organ for FGF23 in rats. *J. Clin. Invest*, 117:4003-4008, 2007.

[12] Mannstadt M, Jüppner H, Gardella TJ. Receptors for PTH and PTHrP: their biological importance and functional properties. *Am. J. Physiol.* 1999 Nov;277(5 Pt 2):F665-75.

[13] Brown EM. Extracellular Ca2+ sensing, regulation of parathyroid cell function, and role of Ca2+ and other ions as extracellular (first) messengers. *Physiol. Rev.* 1991 Apr;71(2):371-411.

[14] Brown EM, MacLeod R J, Extracellular calcium sensing and extracellular calcium signaling. *J. Physiol. Rev.* 2001;81:239-297.

[15] Schömig M, Ritz E. Management of disturbed calcium metabolism in uraemic patients: 1. Use of vitamin D metabolites. *Nephrol. Dial. Transplant.* 2000;15 Suppl 5:18-24.

[16] Denda M, Finch J, Brown AJ, Nishii Y, Kubodera N, Slatopolsky E. 1,25-dihydroxyvitamin D3 and 22-oxacalcitriol prevent the decrease in vitamin D receptor content in the parathyroid glands of uremic rats. Kidney Int. 1996 Jul;50(1):34-9.

[17] Murray TM, Rao LG, Divieti P, Bringhurst FR. Parathyroid hormone secretion and action: evidence for discrete receptors for the carboxyl-terminal region and related biological actions of carboxyl- terminal ligands. *Endocr. Rev.* 2005 Feb;26(1):78-113.

[18] Dambacher MA, Fischer JA, Hunziker WH, Born W, Moran J, Roth HR, Delvin EE, Glorieux FH 1979 Distribution of circulating immunoreactive components of parathyroid hormone in normal subjects and in patients with primary and secondary hyperparathyroidism: the role of the kidney and of the serum calcium concentration. *Clin. Sci.* (Lond) 57:435–443.

[19] Donadio C, Ardini M, Lucchesi A, Donadio E, Cantor T. Parathyroid hormone and large related C-terminal fragments increase at different rates with worsening of renal function in chronic kidney disease patients. A possible indicator of bone turnover status? *Clin. Nephrol.* 2007 Mar;67(3):131-9.

[20] Bringhurst FR, Stern AM, Yotts M, Mizrahi N, Segre GV, Potts Jr JT. Peripheral metabolism of PTH: fate of biologically active amino terminus in vivo. *Am. J. Physiol.* 255:E886–E893, 1988.

[21] Lepage R, Roy L, Brossard JH, Rousseau L, Dorais C, Lazure C, et al. Non-(1–84) circulating parathyroid hormone (PTH) fragment interferes significantly with intact PTH commercial assay measurements in uremic samples. *Clin. Chem.* 1998;44:805-809.

[22] Inaba M, Nakatsuka K, Imanishi Y, Watanabe M, Mamiya Y, Ishimura E, Nishizawa Y. Technical and clinical characterization of the Bio-PTH (1-84) immunochemiluminometric assay and comparison with a second-generation assay for parathyroid hormone. *Clin. Chem.* 2004 Feb;50(2):385-90. Epub 2003 Dec 18.

[23] Koller H, Zitt E, Staudacher G, Neyer U, Mayer G, Rosenkranz AR. Variable parathyroid hormone(1-84)/carboxylterminal PTH ratios detected by 4 novel parathyroid hormone assays. *Clin. Nephrol.* 2004 May;61(5):337-43.

[24] Hsu H, Lacey DL, Dunstan CR, Solovyev I, Colombero A, Timms E, Tan HL, Elliott G, Kelley MJ, Sarosi I, Wang L, Xia XZ, Elliott R, Chiu L, Black T, Scully S, Capparelli C, Morony S, Shimamoto G, Bass MB, Boyle WJ. Tumor necrosis factor receptor family member RANK mediates osteoclast differentiation and activation induced by osteoprotegerin ligand. *Proc. Natl. Acad. Sci. U S A.* 1999 Mar 30;96(7):3540-5.

[25] Hulter HN, Peterson JC. Acid-base homeostasis during chronic PTH excess in humans. Kidney Int. 1985 Aug;28(2):187-92.

[26] Horiuchi N, Caulfield M P, Fisher JE, Goldman ME, McKee RL, Reagan JE, Levy JJ, Nutt RF, Rodan SB, Schofield TL, Clemens TL, Rosenblatt M. Similarity of synthetic peptide from human tumour to parathyroid hormone in vivo and in vitro. *Science* 238:1566–1568. 1987.

[27] Huang Z., Chen Y., Pratt S., Chen T.-H., Bambino T., Nissenson R., Shoback D.(1996) The NH2-terminal region of the third intracellular loop of the parathyroid hormone (PTH)/PTH-related peptide receptor is critical for coupling to cAMP and inositol phosphate/Ca2+ signal transduction pathways. *J. Biol. Chem.* 271:33382–33389.

[28] Datta NS, Abou-Samra AB. PTH and PTHrP signaling in osteoblasts. *Cell Signal.* 2009 Aug;21(8):1245-54. Epub 2009 Feb 26.

[29] Jones G, Strugnell SA, DeLuca HF. Current understandings of the molecular actions of Vitamin-D. *Physiological Reviews.* 1998; 78 (4), 1193-1231.

[30] Muff R, Born W, Fischer JA. Calcitonin, calcitonin gene-related peptide, adrenomedullin and amylin: homologous peptides, separate receptors and overlapping biological actions. *Eur. J. Endocrinol.* 133:17-20, 1995.

[31] Singer FR, Melvin KE, Mills BG. Acute effects of calcitonin on osteoclasts in man. *Clin. Endocrinol.* (Oxf). 1976;5 Suppl:333S-340S.

[32] Cochran M, Peacock M, Sachs G, Nordin BE. Renal effects of calcitonin. *Br. Med. J.* 1970 Jan 17;1(5689):135-7.

[33] Root AW, Harrison HE. Recent advances in calcium metabolism. I. Mechanisms of calcium homeostasis. *J. Pediatr.* 1976 Jan;88(1):1-18.

[34] Rutecki PA. Neuronal excitability: voltage-dependent currents and synaptic transmission. *J. Clin. Neurophysiol.* 1992 Apr;9(2):195-211.

[35] Deluca HF. The vitamin D story: a collaborative effort of basic science and clinical medicine.FASEB J. 1988 Mar 1; 2(3):224-36. Review.

[36] Cheah WK, Arici C, Ituarte PH, siperstein AE, Duh QY, Clark OH. Complications of neck dissection for thyroid cancer. *World J. Surg.* 2002 Aug;26(8):1013-6, 2002.

[37] Pattou F, Combemale F, Fabre S, Carnaille B, Decoulx M, Wemeau JL, Racadot A, Proye C. Hypocalcemia following thyroid surgery: incidence and prediction of outcome. *World J. Surg.* 1998 Jul;22(7):718-24.

[38] Asari R, Passler C, Kaczirek K, scheuba C, Niderle B. Hypoparathyroidism after total thyroidectomy: a prospective study. *Arch. Surg.* 143(2): 132-7, 2008.
[39] Roh JL, Park JY, Park CI. Prevention of postoperative hypocalcemia with routine oral calcium and vitamin D supplements in patients with differentiated papillary thyroid carcinoma undergoing total thyroidectomy plus central neck dissection. *Cancer.* 2009 Jan 15;115(2):251-8.
[40] Falko JM, Bush CA, Tzagournis M, Thomas FB. Case report. Congestive heart failure complicating the hungry bone syndrome. *Am. J. Med. Sci.* 1976 Jan-Feb;271(1):85-9.
[41] Brasier AR, Nussbaum SR. Hungry bone syndrome: clinical and biochemical predictors of its occurrence after parathyroid surgery. *Am. J. Med.* 1988 Apr;84(4):654-60.
[42] Rude RK, Oldham SB, Singer FR. Functional hypoparathyroidism and parathyroid hormone end-organ resistance in human magnesium deficiency. *Clin. Endocrinol.* (Oxf). 1976 May;5(3):209-24.
[43] Blizzard RM, Chee D, Davis W. The incidence of parathyroid and other antibodies in the sera of patients with idiopathic hypoparathyroidism. *Clin. Exp. Immunol.* Apr;1(2):119-28, 1966.
[44] Brown EM. Anti-parathyroid and anti-calcium sensing receptor antibodies in autoimmune hypoparathyroidism. *Endocrinol. Metab. Clin. North Am.* 2009 Jun;38(2):437-45.
[45] Podkrajsek KT, Milenković T, Odink RJ, Claasen-van der Grinten HL, Bratanic N, Hovnik T, Battelino T.Detection of a complete autoimmune regulator gene deletion and two additional novel mutations in a cohort of patients with atypical phenotypic variants of autoimmune polyglandular syndrome type 1. *Eur. J. Endocrinol.* Nov;159(5):633-9. 2008.
[46] Egbuna OI, Brown EM. Hypercalcaemic and hypocalcaemic conditions due to calcium-sensing receptor mutations. *Best Pract. Res. Clin. Rheumatol.* 2008 Mar;22(1):129-48.
[47] Pollak MR, Brown EM, Estep HL, et al. 1994 Autosomal dominant hypocalcaemia caused by a Ca(2+)-sensing receptor gene mutation. *Nat. Genet.* 8:303–307.
[48] Hirai H, Nakajima S, Miyauchi A, Nishimura K, Shimizu N, Shima M, Michigami T, Ozono K, Okada S. A novel activating mutation (C129S) in the calcium-sensing receptor gene in a Japanese family with autosomal dominant hypocalcaemia. *J. Hum. Genet.* 2001;46(1):41-4.
[49] Nagase T, Murakami T, Tsukada T, Kitamura R, Chikatsu N, Takeo H, Takata N, Yasuda H, Fukumoto S, Tanaka Y, Nagata N, Yamaguchi K, Akatsu T, Yamamoto M. A family of autosomal dominant hypocalcaemia with a positive correlation between serum calcium and magnesium: identification of a novel gain of function mutation (Ser(820)Phe) in the calcium-sensing receptor. *J. Clin. Endocrinol. Metab.*;87(6):2681-7, 2002 Jun.
[50] Mancilla EE, De Luca F, Ray K, Winer KK, Fan GF, Baron J. A Ca(2+)-sensing receptor mutation causes hypoparathyroidism by increasing receptor sensitivity to Ca2+ and maximal signal transduction. *Pediatr. Res.* 1997 Oct;42(4):443-7.
[51] Chikatsu N, Watanabe S, Takeuchi Y, Muraosa Y, Sasaki S, Oka Y, Fukumoto S, Fujita T.A family of autosomal dominant hypocalcaemia with an activating mutation of calcium-sensing receptor gene. *Endocr. J.* 2003 Feb;50(1):91-6.

[52] Kar PS, Ogoe B, Poole R, Meeking D. Di-George syndrome presenting with hypocalcaemia in adulthood: two case reports and a review. *J. Clin. Pathol.* 2005 Jun;58(6):655-7.

[53] Hasegawa T, Hasegawa Y, Aso T, Koto S, Nagai T, Tsuchiya Y, Kim KC, Ohashi H, Wakui K, Fukushima Y. HDR syndrome (hypoparathyroidism, sensorineural deafness, renal dysplasia) associated with del(10)(p13). *Am. J. Med. Genet.* 1997 Dec 31;73(4):416-8.

[54] Tonelli AR, Kosuri K, Wei S, Chick D. Seizures as the first manifestation of chromosome 22q11.2 deletion syndrome in a 40-year old man: a case report. *J. Med. Case Reports*. 2007 Dec 3;1:167.

[55] Albright F, Burnett CH, Smith PH, Parson W 1942 Pseudohypoparathyroidism—an example of "Seabright-Bantam syndrome". *Endocrinology* 30:922–932.

[56] Weinstein LS, Yu S, Warner DR, Liu J: Endocrine manifestations of stimulatory G protein alpha-subunit mutations and the role of genomic imprinting. *Endocr. Rev.* 2001;22:675–705.

[57] Bastepe M, Jüppner H.GNAS locus and pseudohypoparathyroidism. *Horm. Res.* 2005;63(2):65-74.

[58] Bastepe M, Jüppner H: Pseudohypoparathyroidism: New insights into an old disease. *Endocrinol. Metab. Clin. North Am.* 2000;29:569–589.

[59] Ozbey N, Erbil Y, Ademoğlu E, Ozarmağan S, Barbaros U, Bozbora A. Correlations between vitamin D status and biochemical/clinical and pathological parameters in primary hyperparathyroidism. *World J. Surg*. 2006 Mar;30(3):321-6.

[60] Grey A, Lucas J, Horne A, Gamble G, Davidson JS, Reid IR. Vitamin D repletion in patients with primary hyperparathyroidism and coexistent vitamin D insufficiency. *J. Clin. Endocrinol. Metab.* 2005 Apr;90(4):2122-6.

[61] Winer KK, Ko CW, Reynolds JC, Dowdy K, Keil M, Peterson D, Gerber LH, McGarvey C, Cutler GB Jr. Long-term treatment of hypoparathyroidism: a randomized controlled study comparing parathyroid hormone-(1-34) versus calcitriol and calcium. *J. Clin. Endocrinol. Metab.* 2003 Sep;88(9):4214-20.

[62] Rubin MR, Sliney J Jr, McMahon DJ, Silverberg SJ, Bilezikian JP. Therapy of hypoparathyroidism with intact parathyroid hormone. Osteoporos Int. 2010 Nov;21(11):1927-34. Epub 2010 Jan 22.

[63] Dent DM, Miller JL, Klaff L, Barron J. The incidence and causes of hypercalcaemia. *Postgrad. Med. J.* 1987 Sep;63(743):745-50.

[64] Deftos, LJ: Hypercalcemia in malignant and inflammatory diseases. Endocrinology and Metabolism Clinics of North America 31:1-18, 2002.

[65] Brown EM. Physiology and pathophysiology of the extracellular calcium-sensing receptor. *Am. J. Med.* 1999 Feb;106(2):238-53.

[66] Martin TJ, Suva LJ. Parathyroid Hormone-related Protein in hypercalcaemia of malignancy. *Clin. Endocrinol*; 31(63): 1-647, 1989.

[67] Chen L, Dinh TA and Haque A. Small Cell Carcinoma of the Ovary With Hypercalcemia and Ectopic Parathyroid Hormone Production. *Arch. Pathol. and Lab. Med*:, Vol. 129, No. 4, pp. 531-533. April 2005.

[68] Yoshimoto K, Yamasaki R, Sakai H, Tezuka U, Takahashi M, Iizuka M, Sekiya T, Saito s. Ectopic production of parathyroid hormone by small cell lung cancer in a patient with hypercalcemia. *J. Clin. Endocrinol. metab*. 68(5): 976-81, 1989.

In: Parathyroid: Anatomy, Functions and Disorders
Editor: James Kirkby-Bott
ISBN: 978-1-62100-765-4

Chapter IV

The Effect of Parathyroid Hormone on Bone

Marina Komrakova, Stephan Sehmisch, Klaus Stuermer, and Ewa K Stuermer
Department of Trauma Surgery and Reconstructive Surgery,
University of Goettingen, Robert-Koch, Goettingen, Germany

Abstract

Parathyroid hormone (PTH) plays a central role in the regulation of calcium and phosphate homeostasis. PTH acts directly increasing renal calcium reabsorption and phosphate excretion and indirectly enhancing intestinal calcium absorption. Continuous exposure to exogenous PTH causes an increase in bone resorption, whereas, bone formation is stimulated when PTH is delivered intermittently. There are two areas of research with intermittent PTH application - improvement of bone tissue and the use of PTH to enhance bone repair after fracture. Currently, human parathyroid hormone (hPTH 1-84) and its analog, recombinant hPTH 1-34, are being used for treatment of severe osteoporosis in humans. However, this treatment has significant limitations related to its daily subcutaneous administration and high costs. Little data exist on the effect of PTH treatments of different durations and regimes. The chapter is focused on the effect of PTH on bone tissue either intact or injured in healthy or osteoporotic subjects applied at different regimes and durations.

Evaluation of the lumbar vertebral region is also extremely important because of its high clinical relevance in the treatment of osteoporosis. In a series of experiments, three-month old rats developed osteoporotic changes after ovariectomy during 8 weeks, healthy rats were left intact. Thereafter, all rats underwent bilateral transverse osteotomy in tibia metaphysis (day 0) and were treated with PTH applied at different regimes.

After 35 post-osteotomy days their lumbar spine was analyzed. The first lumbar vertebral body (L1) was used for histological analysis, L2 for computed tomographic (CT) analysis, L3 was ashed and L4 was used for biomechanical testing. In the first trial, five-week daily PTH treatment improved cortical and cancellous bone parameters in lumbar spine in ovariectomy induced osteopenic rats (Ovx).

In trial II, healthy rats were treated 5 times per week either for up to 35 or 28 days. Both PTH treatments improved bone parameters, however, the effect was less when PTH was applied for a shorter period. In trial III, rats were divided into 7 groups: 1) healthy; 2) Ovx; 3) healthy treated with PTH 5 times from day 7 after osteotomy onward (PTH 5x/w 7-35d); 4) "Ovx PTH 5x/w 7-35d"; 5) Ovx PTH every other day (qod) 7-35; 6) "Ovx PTH 5x/w 14-35d"; 7) Ovx PTH 5x/w 14-28d". Single dosage of PTH was 40μg/kg BW. Biomechanical properties improved after PTH treatment in all rats. Yield load improvement was in healthy: 191 to 224 N/mm (PTH 5x/w 7-35d); in Ovx: 148 to 186 N/mm (PTH 5x/w 7-35d). However, the improvement was less when PTH was applied every other day and for a shorter period. Trabecular width increased after PTH treatment (5x/w 7-35d) in healthy from 8.3 to 9.1 μm, in Ovx from 7.5 to 9.3 μm, in Ovx PTH qod 7-35d, PTH 14-35d and PTH 14-28d was 8.6, 5.3, 8.3 μm. BMD increased after all PTH treatments in both healthy and Ovx rats.

Comparing the response of lumbar spine and osteotomized tibia, the differences were detected. It appears that duration and frequency of PTH administration are important parameters when PTH applied for treatment of lumbar spine. When PTH applied to improve tibia healing, the frequency is less important. Furthermore, the improvements observed in lumbar spine of both estrogen deficient and healthy rats were similar. For osteotomy healing PTH stimulation was more effective in healthy than in Ovx rats.

The findings of these studies may show up a potential, although as yet unproven, perspective for therapeutic treatment of osteoporotic patients with or without bone fracture as well as in healthy patients with retarded fracture healing. Further studies are also needed to investigate possible synergistic effect with other anti-osteoporotic agents and the changes occurred after cessation of PTH treatment.

Introduction

Naturally produced parathyroid hormone (PTH) is an 84 amino acid peptide (1-84) secreted by the parathyroid glands. PTH playes a major role in regulation of the concentration of calcium, phosphate, and active vitamin-D metabolites in blood and cellular activity in bone through its effect on bone, kidneys and intestine [1]. PTH enhances the release of calcium from the large reservoir contained in the bones in 2 ways [2]. The rapid phase brings about a rise in serum calcium within minutes and appears to occur at the level of the osteoblasts and osteocytes. These cells form an interconnected network known as the osteocytic membrane overlying the bone matrix, but with a small layer of interposed fluid termed bone fluid. When PTH binds to receptors on these cells, the osteocytic membrane pumps calcium ions from the bone fluid into the extracellular fluid. The slow phase of bone resorption occurs over several days. First, osteoclasts are activated to digest formed bone, and second, osteoclasts are proliferated. Since mature osteoclasts lack PTH membrane receptors, activation and proliferation appears to be stimulated by cytokines released by activated osteoblasts and osteocytes or by differentiation of immature osteoclast precursors that possess PTH and vitamin D receptors [2]. As bone is resorbed both calcium and phosphate are released. The response to PTH by the kidney is to enhance phosphate excretion while promoting calcium reabsorption in the renal tubular system [2]. This increases calcium concentration in blood. Another important function of PTH is enhancement of calcium absorption in the intestine by increasing the conversion of 25-hydroxy-vitamin D to its most active metabolite, 1,25-dihydroxy-vitamin D, activating the enzyme 1-hydroxylase in the kidney. Feedback inhibition of PTH release occurs primarily by direct effect of serum calcium level on the activity of parathyroid gland [2]. Thus, PTH increases serum calcium levels by enhancing gastrointestinal calcium absorption, increases renal calcium reabsorption, liberates calcium from the skeleton in response to systemic needs and participate in the regulation of vitamin-D metabolism [3]. The normal physiological role of PTH on skeletal homeostasis, when secreted endogenously, is more complex but probably serves to regulate bone remodeling rather than overall skeletal mass [4].

It has been generally assumed that the main biological activity of PTH resides in N-terminal sequence 1-34, now named teriparatide [4] [5], although it is possible that C-terminal fragments may have discrete biological properties [6]. It has been determined that PTH (1-34), can reproduce the major biological actions attributed to full-length PTH, including activation of adenyl cyclase both in bone and kidney cells, increased urinary excretion of cyclic adenosine monophosphate and phosphate in rats, and elevation of blood calcium in rats, dogs and chicks [5].

PTH has varying effects on bone tissue depending on the mode of administration. Chronic elevation of PTH levels as in hyperparathyroidism increases bone resorption leading to bone loss [7], whereas, daily (intermittent) administration of PTH stimulates new bone formation [8]. Molecular and cellular mechanisms by which intermittent administration produce anabolic effects are of considerable interest, however, they are not completely understood so far [9] [10]. Intermittent PTH administration directly activates survival signaling in osteoblasts, attenuates osteoblast apoptosis, thereby increasing osteoblast number, bone formation rate and bone mass, but does not affect osteoclast number [9]. These effects of intermittent PTH may explain why PTH therapy reverses bone loss in most osteoporotic individuals regardless of the underlying pathophysiology [10]. Osteoporosis is a progressive systemic skeletal disease characterized by low bone mass and micro-architectural deterioration of bone tissue, leading to enhanced fragility and risk of fracture. Women are at greater risk of developing of osteoporosis as bone loss is accelerated following the menopause due to estrogen deficiency. Nevertheless, other factors such as nutritional, genetic and lifestyle factors also play a role in the development of osteoporosis. PTH represents a new class of anabolic agent for the treatment of severe osteoporosis. It is unlike other therapies to manage osteoporosis, which act mainly by reducing bone turnover and preserving, rather than improving skeletal architecture [4]. Daily administration of parathyroid hormone peptides (1-84 and 1-34) reduces vertebral fracture risk and non-vertebral fracture incidence in postmenopausal women with osteoporosis [8] [11]. However, treatment with PTH has significant limitations related to its daily subcutaneous administration and high costs. Little data exists on the effect of PTH treatments of different durations and regimes. In animal based studies, various regimes of PTH administration were used, however, the results obtained from these trials show variation to the extent that it becomes difficult to reach a definitive conclusion. [12] [13].

There are several researchable areas with intermittent PTH application but two areas of research are pronouncedly important including improvement of bone tissue and prevention of fracture and the use of PTH to enhance bone repair after fracture [1]. This chapter is focused on the effect of PTH on bone tissue either intact or injured in healthy or osteoporotic organism subjects applied at different regimes and durations.

PTH and Bone Tissue

Two PTH analogues, teriparatide (Forsteo) recombinant human PTH (1-34) and Preotact, recombinant human PTH (1-84) are available for treatment of postmenopausal women with osteoporosis and for men with primary or hypogonadal osteoporosis who are both at high risk for fracture [14] 15]. The molecular effects of intermittent PTH application are multiple, such as: activation of bone cells on quiescent surfaces to function as osteoblasts, stimulation of differentiation of preosteoblast to osteoblast, and prolongation of life span of mature osteoblasts [16] [17]. Thus, intermittent PTH application leads to an increase in osteoblastic number and function, thereby leading to a rapid increase in skeletal mass. PTH daily injections improve skeletal microarchitecture, bone strength, and bone mass, which, in turn, may reduce the risk of fracture [11] [16] [17] [18]. Intermittent PTH restores structure of trabecular bone [19] [20] in osteoporosis and also has a positive effect on cortical bone. [21] [22]. Teriparatide has been shown to reduce the risk of fracture in postmenopausal women with osteoporosis [11].

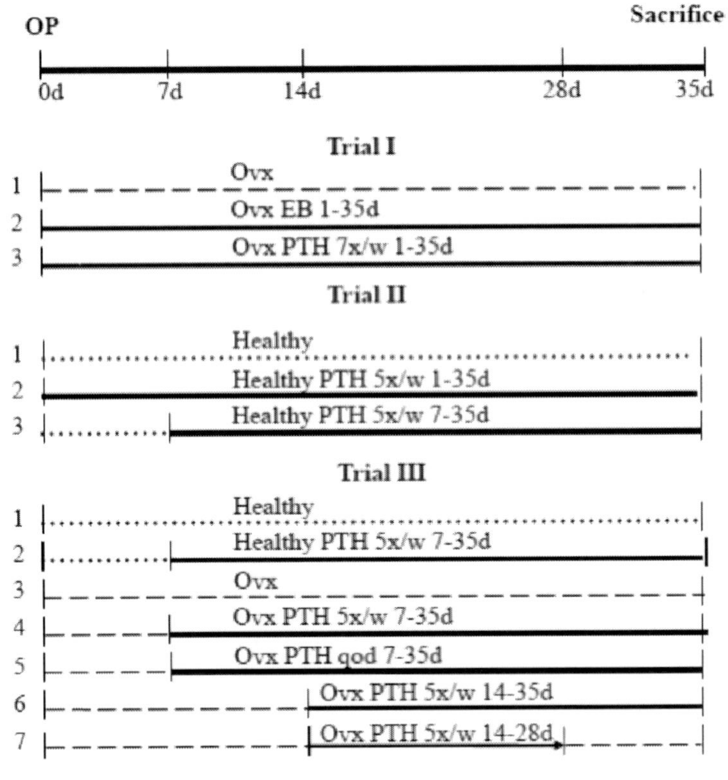

Figure 1. Schematic flowchart of 3 trials.

Daily treatment with teriparatide 20μg or 40 μg for 18 months increased bone mineral density (BMD) by 9% and 13 % at the lumbar spine and by 3% and 6% at the hip. New vertebral fracture occurred in 14% of women in the placebo group and in 5% and 4% of the women in 20μg and 40μg PTH treated groups respectively. The authors concluded that the 40μg dose of PTH increased bone mineral density more than the 20 μg dose but there was no significant difference in effect on the risk of fracture and the 40μg dose was more likely to produce side effects [11]. Teriparatide applied for 19 months significantly increased trabecular bone volume and trabecular connectivity in postmenopausal women [22]. PTH increased lumbar spine BMD in all studies, at several dosages, for any duration, in different clinical situations, and in combination with multiple agents [23]. The femoral neck responded to PTH treatments variously either showing no changes in BMD, increasing BMD or only partly prevented bone loss [23]. Intermittent PTH administration by daily injections is approved as the first form of osteoporosis therapy that is anabolic to bone tissue, reverses bone deficit and reduces the incidence of fracture.

A regime of PTH administration used in animal studies varied from a daily administration to 3, or 5 times a week or even once a week [12] [13] making comparisons difficult. Furthermore, bone response to PTH is more enhanced in the presence of gonadal hormones compared to that in hormone deficient subjects [24] [25].

To explore more efficient use of PTH treatment, the effect of PTH applied at different regimes was studied in healthy and ovariectomy induced osteopenic rats. All rats (5 months of age) underwent bilateral transverse osteotomy in the tibia metaphysis on day 0 as described in the "PTH and bone repair" section. Data on bone healing has been published previously [25]. Further studies have focused on the lumbar spine because of its high clinical relevance in the treatment of osteoporosis. The first lumbar vertebral body (L1) was used for histological analysis, L2 for computed tomographic (fpVCT) analysis, L3 was ashed, while L4 was used for biomechanical tests. In the first trial, ovariectomized (Ovx) rats after developing osteoporotic changes over a 2 month period were divided into 3 groups: rats treated with PTH seven times a week (7x/w, 40 μg/kg BW, 1-35d), with oral estradiol-17β-benzoate (0.4 mg/kg BW, 1-35d) or left untreated (Fig. 4.1, Trial I). After 35 days, PTH enhanced the serum level of osteocalcin (46 ng/mL) compared to that in untreated OVX rats (18 ng/mL). In estrogen treated rats osteocalcin (Oc) was at the lowest level (5 ng/mL). Biomechanical properties of lumbar vertebral body were improved solely after PTH treatment, whereas, histological studies revealed improvement of bone parameters after both PTH and estrogen treatments, though the effect of estrogen was less pronounced [26]. In a follow-up study, the effect of PTH on the lumbar vertebral body was studied in healthy rats. Five-month old rats were divided into 3 groups, 12 rats in each (Figure 4.1, Trial II). The Group 1 was left untreated, while Group 2 and 3 were treated with PTH 5 times a week (40 μg/kg) during either 35 days or 28 days (1-35d, 7-35d). Serum Oc level, total BMD, trabecular parameters increased significantly after both PTH treatments (Table 4.1). Biomechanical properties and ash weight increased after PTH treatments, reaching a significant level in the group treated with PTH for 35 days. PTH treatment resulted in an increase in cortical width, though to a lesser extent in the "PTH 7-35d" group. Serum alkaline phosphatase (Alp) was not sensitive to PTH (Table 4.1). The relative mRNA expression of osteoblast marker, Oc was higher in the "PTH 5x/w 7-35" group than in the other 2 groups (Figure 4.2). Expression of the osteoclast marker, acid phosphatase 5 (Acp 5) increased significantly after both PTH treatments. The relative mRNA expression of osteoblast marker, Oc was higher in the "PTH 5x/w 7-35" group than in the other 2 groups (Figure 4.2). Expression of the osteoclast marker, acid phosphatase 5 (Acp 5) increased significantly after both PTH treatments.

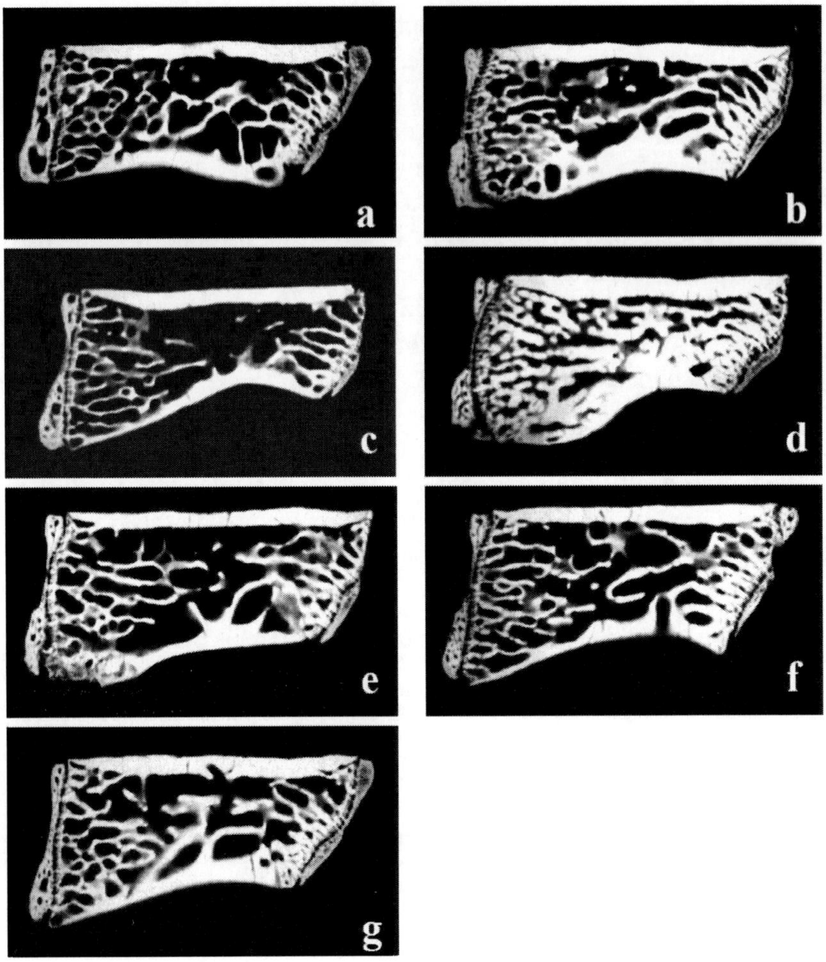

Figure 2. Box plot illustrating relative expression level of (a) Alp, (b) Oc, (c) Igf-1, (d) Acp 5, (e) Rankl, (f) Opg genes in treatment groups (1) "healthy", (2) "healthy PTH 5x/w 1-35d", (3) "healthy PTH 5x/w 7-35d" calculated using $2^{-\Delta\Delta CT}$ method (Livak and Schmittgen 2001) relative to gene expression in an untreated healthy group (at least 9 replications per group). Medians with different letters differ significantly (P0.05, Kruskal-Wallis-test) (Trial II).

The mRNA expression of Alp, Igf-1, Rankl and Opg did not change by PTH treatment. Subsequent to the above trials further studies were done to compare the efficacy of different regimes of PTH administration. Three-month old rats developed osteopenia during 8 weeks after ovariectomy; healthy rats were left intact (Figure 1, Trial III). After the osteotomy was performed, rats were divided into 7 groups (12 rats in each) 1) healthy; 2) healthy treated with PTH 5 times per week during 28 days (PTH 5x/w, 7-35d); 3) Ovx; 4) "Ovx PTH 5x/w, 7-35d"; 5) Ovx PTH every other day (qod), 7-35d; 6) "Ovx PTH 5x/w, 14-35d"; 7) Ovx PTH 5x/w, 14-28d". Single dosage of PTH was 40 μg/kg BW. After 35 postoperative days the lumbar spine was analyzed. The results showed that biomechanical properties, bone density, cortical and trabecular width were improved after PTH treatment in both healthy and Ovx rats (Table 2).

Table 1. Serum analyses, biomechanical, ashing, fpVCT and histological analyses of lumbar vertebral bodies in healthy rats either untreated or treated with PTH at different regimes. At least 11 replications per treatment group were done. Data are shown as means and standard error of the mean (Trial II)

Parameters	Healthy		Healthy PTH 5x/w 1-35d		Healthy PTH 5x/w 7-35d	
	Mean	SEM	Mean	SEM	Mean	SEM
Serum analyses						
Oc (µg/L)	23^{a}	2	37^{b}	3	37^{b}	3
Alp (U/L)	43	3	51	3	48	3
Biomechanics (L4)						
Stiffness (N/mm)	141^{a}	10	276^{b}	27	199^{a}	16
Yield load (N)	249	18	291	10	270	15
Fmax	255	18	298	10	285	13
Ashing (L3)						
Ash/Volume (mg/mm^{3})	2.06^{a}	0.08	2.51^{b}	0.15	2.34^{ab}	0.10
fpVCT (L2)						
Total BMD (mg/cm^{3})	444^{a}	8	489^{b}	4	495^{b}	5
Histology (L1)						
Ct.width (mm)	0.38^{a}	0.01	0.47^{b}	0.01	0.43^{c}	0.01
Tr. width (µm)	5.8^{a}	0.2	7.3^{b}	0.2	7.1^{b}	0.2
Tr. Dn (n/mm^{2})	5.2^{a}	0.2	5.7^{b}	0.1	5.8^{b}	0.1

^{abc} Within row means with different superscripts differ (P 0.05, Scheffé-test).

Table 2. Serum analyses, biomechanical, ashing, fpVCT and histological analyses of lumbar vertebral bodies in healthy or Ovx rats either untreated or treated with PTH at different regimes. At least 9 replications per treatment group were done. Data are shown as means and standard error of the mean (Trial III)

Parameters	Healthy		Healthy PTH 5x/w 7-35d		Ovx		Ovx PTH 5x/w 7-35d		Ovx PTH 3x/w 7-35d		Ovx PTH 5x/w 14-35d		Ovx PTH 5x/w 14-28d	
Serum analyses														
Oc (µg/L)	15^{a}	2	23^{bc}	2	18^{ab}	2	33^{d}	2	37^{d}	3	24^{bc}	4	16^{a}c	3
Alp (U/L)	41^{ab}	7	54^{ab}	6	60^{ac}	6	60^{a} 4		74^{c}	7	40^{b}	7	51^{ab}	10
Biomechanics (L4)														
Stiffness (N/mm)	133^{ab}	9	188^{c}	17	115^{b}	6	145^{ab}	13	157^{ac}	13	142^{ab}	11	139^{ab} 8	
Yield load (N)	191^{ac}	12	224c	13	148^{b}	7	186^{ad}	13	156^{bd}	10	210^{ac}	12	181^{ad}	13
Fmax (N)	196^{a}	13	269^{c}	10	155^{b}	7	229^{a}	16	203^{a}	9	228^{a}	9	215^{a}	13
Ashing (L3)														
Ash/Volume (mg/mm^{3})	1.94	0.10	2.13	0.09	1.72	0.18	1.92	0.08	1.95	0.06	2.09	0.11	2.13	0.09
fpVCT (L2)														
BMD (mg/cm3)	491^{a}	9	561^{b}	12	435^{c} 4		507^{a}	8	474^{a}	11	499^{a}	6	482^{a}	6
Histology (L1)														
Ct.width (mm)	0.25^{a}	0.01	0.29^{c}	0.01	0.24^{a}	0.01	0.28^{cd}	0.01	0.27^{bd}	0.01	0.25^{a}	0.01	0.26^{b}	0.01
Tr. width (µm)	8.3^{a}	0.2	9.1^{c}	0.1	7.5^{b}	0.1	9.3^{c}	0.1	8.6^{a}	0.1	8.3^{a}	0.2	8.3^{a}	0.1
Tr. Dn (n.Nd/mm^{2})	15.6^{a}	0.4	15.5^{a}	0.6	11.6^{d}	0.3	13.9^{c}	0.6	12.2^{bd}	0.3	13.1^{cb}	0.3	12.9^{cb}	0.3

^{abcd} Within row means with different superscripts differ (P 0.05, Scheffé-test).

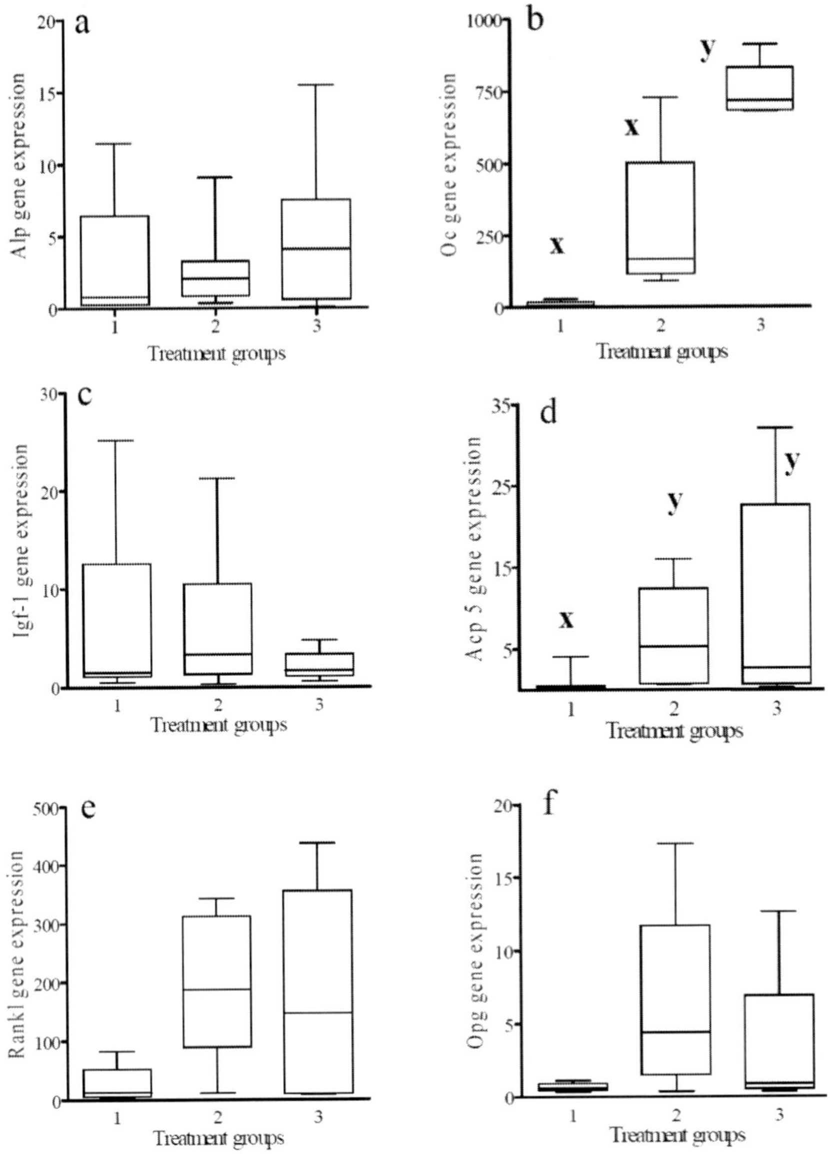

Figure 3. Image of microradiographed sagittal sections of second vertebral body made 35 days after tibia osteotomy in treatment groups: (a) healthy, (b) "healthy PTH 5x/w 7-35d", (c) Ovx, (d) Ovx PTH 5x/w 7-35d", (e) "Ovx PTH qod 7-35d", (f) "Ovx PTH 5x/w 14-35d", (g) "Ovx PTH 5x/w 14-28d" (Trial III). In Ovx rats, deteriorated bone structure is determined (c); PTH (7-35d) results in a denser trabecular network and thicker cortical and trabecular structures (b, d); PTH applied with less frequency and for a shorter period has less effect on bone (e, f, g).

The BMD was higher in PTH treated rats irrespectively of estrogen status and PTH administration regimes. However, PTH treatment was less effective for cortical and trabecular bone parameters when it was applied for a shorter period (14-35d and 14-28d) or with less frequency (qod 7-35d) (Table 4.2, Figure 4.3). Ash weight did not differ between the groups (Table 4.2). Parathyroid hormone improved lumbar spine properties depending on duration and frequency of the treatment in both estrogen deficient and healthy rats.

PTH and Bone Repair

Whereas parathyroid hormone is approved for treatment of severe osteoporosis in humans, the effect of PTH on bone healing is still underestimated. PTH has potential as a systemic anabolic agent for enhancement of bone healing without operative intervention. PTH administered after operative intervention may facilitate bone repair ensuring patients have a more rapid return to an active life style.

Recent reports have shown that intermittent treatment with PTH facilitates bone healing promoting chondrogenesis and osteogenesis in experimental animals [1] [27]. The favorable effect of PTH on bone healing does not require previous stimulation of bone resorption induced by ovariectomy or orchidectomy [1]. An effect of PTH on fracture healing was investigated in a rat diaphyseal femur fracture model stabilized using an intramedullary pin by several recent studies [12] [28] [29] [30] [31].

[28] examined the effect of daily PTH (1-34) administration (80μg/kg) on fracture healing in the femur of intact 3-month old male rats. Twenty-one days after fracture, the callus area and strength increased significantly in PTH treated rats. [32] studied the effect of daily PTH (1-34) treatment (60 or 200 μg/kg) on unilateral closed tibia shaft fracture fixed with Kirchner wire in 3-month old female rats. The 200 μg/kg PTH dose improved callus properties after 20 and 40 days, whereas, the dose of 60 μg/kg improved healing after 40 days. Both doses steadily augmented the intact contralateral tibia in a dose depending manner. Further, the authors studied the influence of daily PTH (1-34) treatment (200 μg/kg) in 27-month old rats after 3 or 8 weeks of tibia healing [33]. The PTH treatment enhanced fracture strength, callus volume and callus bone mineral content during the healing period.

Nakajima et al. [12], performed a closed femoral fracture in 2-month old male rats. The PTH (1-34) was applied at daily doses of 2, 10, 50 or 100 μg/kg. After 28 and 42 days of healing, callus formation was significantly enlarged after PTH treatment in a dose dependent manner. The minimum effective dose was 10 μg/kg. Further studies using this dose showed increased bone mineral content and density as well as biomechanical properties of fractured femora in treated rats [12]. The expression levels of type I collagen (Col1a1), osteonectin (On), alkaline phosphatase (Alp) and insulin-like growth factor I (Igf-I) mRNA were enhanced in PTH treated rats during the first 4-7 days after fracture. The increased expression of osteocalcin (Oc), Col1a1, Oc, Alp mRNA continued during the later stages of healing (days 14-21), whereas, expression level of Igf-I decreased to the level observed in the untreated group. The authors suggested that PTH enhanced callus formation by the early stimulation of proliferation and differentiation of osteoprogenitor cells, increased production of bone matrix proteins and enhanced osteoclastogenesis during the phase of callus remodeling. The PTH did not change biomechanical properties, bone mass and mRNA expression of genes in intact femora probably because of a low dose of PTH and relatively short time of exposure [12].

Alkhiary et al. [29] compared the effect of daily treatment with 2 doses of PTH (1-34) (5 or 30 μg/kg) on femoral fracture performed in 7 to 9-month old male rats. Treatments were discontinued at 35 days. The results showed that PTH enhanced fracture healing by increasing bone mineral density and biomechanical parameters after 21, 35 and 84 days when given a PTH dose of 30μg/kg. PTH produced a sustained anabolic effect throughout the remodeling phase of fracture healing. The effect of 5μg/kg dose of PTH was less; improving solely bone mineral density after 35 days of healing.

These studies have demonstrated the favorable effect of PTH on osteogenesis in experimental fracture healing. [30] investigated the effect of daily PTH (1-34) treatment (10μg/kg) on chondrogenesis in femoral fracture in 2-month old male rats. PTH increased mRNA expression of SOX-9, COL2A1 and COL10A1 genes during 7 days after fracture resulting in an elevated mesenchymal (chondroprogenitor) cell proliferation and in formation of a larger cartilaginous callus on day 14 after fracture, whereas, on days 21 and 28, the effect of PTH was not revealed. The authors suggested that low-dose PTH did not delay chondrocyte differentiation during fracture healing. In contrast, additional trials showed that higher doses of PTH (400 and 800 μg/kg) may impair maturation of hypertrophic chondrocytes and inhibit replacement of cartilage with bone [30].

Komatsubara et al. [31] reported that treatment with PTH (1-34) at a dose of 30 μg/kg before and after osteotomy performed in midschaft femora in 5-week old female rats accelerated healing process by earlier replacement of woven bone to lamellar bone, increased new cortical shell formation, and increased ultimate load up to 12 weeks after osteotomy. Treatment with PTH only before osteotomy at dose of 30 or 10 μg/kg, and 10 μg/kg before and after osteotomy showed less effect on osteotomy healing.

These results have provided evidence that PTH may enhance fracture healing promoting chondrogenesis and osteogenesis, and accelerating bone remodeling from woven to lamellar bone in healthy experimental animals and only a few studies have examined the efficacy of PTH for impaired fracture healing, e.g. in osteoporotic animals [13] [25] [34]. Osteoporosis has been reported to influence the early, middle and late periods of fracture healing in rats inducing a decrease in mineralized tissue and not well connected microstructure in newly formed callus [35] [36].

Kim and Jahng [34] examined healing of bilateral closed tibia shaft fracture stabilized by intramedullary nailing with Kirschner wires after daily treatment with PTH (1-84) (15 or 150 μg/kg) in 7- month old ovariectomy induced osteopenic rats (Ovx at 4 months of age). After 30 days of healing, it was observed that PTH improved morphometric and mechanical parameters in a dose-dependent manner.

It is known in humans, osteoporotic fractures predominantly occur at the metaphysis of long bones where osteoporotic changes are more pronounced. Testing the effect of PTH on cancellous bone which is most affected by osteoporosis, [13] studied bone healing in the right proximal tibia. Complete mid-sagittal osteotomy from the joint surface to the tibial diaphysis was performed in 7-month old female rats and fixed with cerclage wiring circumferentially. Ovariectomy was performed during osteotomy operation. Sham operated or ovariectomized rats were either treated with PTH (1-34) (100 μg/kg) or given its vehicle (0.1M sodium acetate buffer (pH 7.2) containing 0.1% bovine serum albumin) once a week for 4 weeks [13]. One week after the last injection the rats were euthanized and bilateral tibiae were prepared for histological analyses. PTH increased cancellous bone volume, bone union and rate of proliferating cells at the osteotomy site, and suppressed adipocyte volume in bone marrow in both sham and Ovx rats.

The PTH is usually applied from the day of fracture onward and little is known on the potential of PTH administrated at different stages of bone healing. [25] investigated the effect of PTH (1-34) treatment (40 μg/kg) applied at different regimes on osteotomy healing in healthy and ovariectomy induced osteopenic rats (Ovx at 3 month of age). Using bilateral metaphyseal osteotomy of tibia with plate osteosynthesis [37], after 35 days it was demonstrated that PTH administration from days 1 and 7 after osteotomy improved healing in both osteopenic and healthy rats regardless of application frequency (7, 5 times per week or every other day) being more effective in healthy rats. Administration from day 14 after osteotomy proved to be less effective. Serum osteocalcin level was elevated in PTH treated rats, whereas, serum alkaline phosphatase was found to be not sensitive to PTH treatments. mRNA expression of bone genes in callus was not affected by PTH after 35 days post-osteotomy. The authors concluded that PTH promoted bone healing when it was applied during early stage of healing; stimulation of healing by PTH might be more effective in healthy subjects with unaltered level of gonadal hormones than in estrogen deficient rats.

For practical and statistical reasons, most of the studies are conducted on rat models despite the differences in physiology and bone structure between rat and human. The rats do not have intracortical remodeling. However, [38] studied the effect of PTH on bone healing using a primate model. Adult female Cynomolgus monkeys aged 18-19 years were treated with PTH (1-34) at a dose of 0.75 μg/kg or 7.5 μg/kg. Injection was initiated 3 weeks before experimental fracture and performed twice a week during 26 weeks after osteotomy. Transverse osteotomy was performed at the midshaft of the right femur and fixed tightly with a stainless plate. The PTH treatment of higher dose improved biomechanical properties and enhanced the degree of mineralization of callus. Callus size and porosity decreased and degree of callus mineralization increased after both PTH treatments. PTH accelerated primate fracture healing without affecting structural properties. Since PTH effect on bone is reversed after cessation of treatment [39], some authors investigated the combined therapy of PTH and other osteoporotic agents. Pretreatment with alendronate and PTH or alendronate treatment alone prevented the development of nonunion of osteotomized midschaft femur in estrogen deficient rats [40]. The synergetic effect of PTH and mechanical loading has been shown investigating osteotomy healing of tibia diaphysis in 10-week old male mice [41].

Conclusion

The differences in the response of injured and intact bones may show up a potential, although as yet unproven, perspective for therapeutic treatment of osteoporotic patients with or without bone fracture and also for healthy patients with retarded fracture healing. For the osteoporotic patients, high costs of daily administration of PTH seemed to be justified because the duration and the frequency of PTH applications are important parameters for improvement of bone tissue. When giving PTH to improve bone healing, the frequency is less important. PTH given 7 or 5 times per week or every other day enhances bone repair in animal models. PTH improves vertebral body properties irrespectively of estrogen status, whereas, for tibia healing PTH stimulation is more effective in models with normal estrogen level than in estrogen deficient ones. Presumably, in the injured bone regenerative mechanisms are activated and may interfere with PTH action. There is also concern that the changes in osteoporotic models might blunt the bone healing effects of PTH to some extent. On the other hand, various responses to PTH by different anatomic sites have also been reported in humans [23]. The differences are also revealed analyzing bone gene expression after PTH treatment in a rat model. Whereas, in callus of osteotomized tibia no changes were found in mRNA gene expression 35 days after osteotomy [25], at the same time in lumbar vertebral body, bone formation and bone resorption genes were up-regulated after PTH treatment.

In conclusion it is remarked that PTH may be used to facilitate the healing of bone in healthy as well as in osteoporotic organisms. PTH applied for treatment of osteoporosis is usually administered over a 2-year period. Nevertheless, the anabolic effect of PTH is reversed once the treatment is discontinued. Treatment strategies should, therefore, consider the appropriate post-PTH treatment. Further studies are needed to develop combination therapy of PTH and other anti-osteoporotic agents that may be either given concomitantly or sequentially.

References

[1] Barnes GL, Kakar S, Vora S, Morgan EF, Gerstenfeld LC, Einhorn TA, 2008. Stimulation of fracture-healing with systemic intermittent parathyroid hormone treatment. *J. Bone Joint Surg. Am.* 90(Suppl 1):120-127.

[2] Essig Jr GF, Jameson MJ, Carter WB, Carron JD, 2010. Parathyroid physiology. http://emedicine.medscape.com/article/874690-overview

[3] Jüppner H, Kronenberg HM, 2003. Parathyroid hormone. In: Favus MJ, editor. Primer on the metabolic bone diseases and disorders of mineral metabolism. 5th ed. Washington, DC:American Society for Bone and Mineral Research, P. 117-124.

[4] Hodsman AB, Bauer DC, Dempster DW, Dian L, Hanley DA, Steven TH, Kendler DL, McClung MR, Miller PD, Olszynski WP, Orwoll E, Yuen CK, 2005. Parathyroid hormone and teriparatide for the treatment of osteoporosis: a review of the evidence and suggested quidelines for its use. *Endocr. Rev.* 26, 688-703.

[5] Murray TM, Rao LG, Divieti P, Bringhurst FR, 2005. Parathyroid hormone secretion and action: evidence for discrete receptors for the carboxyl-terminal region and related biological actions of carboxyl-terminal ligands. *Endocr. Rev.* 26, 78-113.

[6] Divieti P, Inomata N, Singh R, Juppner H, Bringhurst FR, 2001. Receptors for the carboxyl-terminal region of PTH (1-84) are highly expressed in osteocytic cells. *Endocrinology* 142, 916-925.

[7] Potts JT, 2005. Parathyroid hormone: past and present. *J. Endocrinol.* 187, 311-325.

[8] Compston JE, 2007. Skeletal actions of intermittent parathyroid hormone: Effects on bone remodeling and structure. *Bone* 40, 1447-1452.

[9] Bellido T, Ali AA, Plotkin LI, Fu Q, Gubrij I, Roberson PK, Weinstein RS, O´Brien CA, Manolagas SC, Jilka RL, 2003. Proteasomal degradation of Runx2 shortens parathyroid hormone-induced anti-apoptotic signaling in osteoblasts. A putative explanation for why intermittent administration is needed for bone anabolism. *J. Biol. Chem.* 278, 50259-50272.

[10] Alkhiary YM, Gerstenfeld LC, Krall E, Westmore M, Sato M, Mitlak BH, Einhorn TA, 2005. Enhancement of experimental fracture-healing by systemic administration of recombinant human parathyroid hormone (PTH 1–34). *Bone Joint Surg. Am.* 87, 731-741.

[11] Andreassen TT, Ejersted C, Oxlund H, 1999. Intermittent parathyroid hormone (1-34) treatment increases callus formation and mechanical strength of healing rat fracture. *J. Bone Miner. Res.* 14, 960-968.

[12] Andreassen TT, Fledelius C, Ejersted C, Oxlund H, 2001. Increases in callus formation and mechanical strength of healing fractures in old rats treated with parathyroid hormone. *Acta Orthop. Scand.* 72, 304-307.

[13] Black DM, Bilezikian JP, Ensrud KE, Greespan SL, Palermo L, Hue T, Lang TF, McGowan JA, Rosen CJ, for the PaTH Study Investigators, 2005. One year alendronate after one year of parathyroid hormone (1-84) for osteoporosis. *N. Engl. J. Med.* 353, 555-565.

[14] Capuzzo KA, Delafuente JC, 2004. Teriparatide for severe osteoporosis. *Ann. Pharmacother.* 38, 294-302.

[15] Crandall C, 2002. Parathyroid hormone for treatment of osteoporosis. *Arch. Intern Med.* 162, 2297-2309.

[16] Dobnig H, Turner RT, 1997. The effects of programmed administration of human parathyroid hormone fragment (1-34) on bone histomorphometry and serum chemistry in rats. *Endocrinology* 138, 4607-4612.

[17] Dobnig H, Turner RT, 1995. Evidence that intermittent treatment with parathyroid hormone increases bone formation in adult rats by activation of bone cell lines. *Endocrinology* 136, 3632-3638.

[18] Gallacher SJ, Dixon T, 2010. Impact of treatments for postmenopausal osteoporosis (bisphosphonates, parathyroid hormone, strontium ranelate, and denosumab) on bone quality:a systematic review. Calcif Tissue Int. DOI 10.1007/s00223-010-9420-x

[19] Gardner MJ, van der Meulen, MCH, Carson J, Zelken J, Ricciardi BF, Wright TM, Lane JM, Bostrom MP, 2007. Role of parathyroid hormone in the mechanosensitivity of fracture healing. *J. Orthop. Res.* 25, 1474-1480.

[20] Gunness M, Hock JM, 1993. Anabolic effect of parathyroid hormone on cancellous and cortical bone histology. *Bone* 14, 277-281.

[21] Hodsman AB, Kisiel M, Adachi JD, Fraher LJ, Watson PH, 2000. Histomorphometric evidence for increased bone turnover without change in cortical thickness or porosity after 2 years of cyclical hPTH (1-34) therapy in women with severe osteoporosis. *Bone* 27, 311-318.

[22] Holzer G, Majeska RJ, Lundy MW, Hartke JR, Einhorn TA, 1999. Parathyroid hormone enhances fracture healing. *Clin. Orthop. Relat. Res.* 366, 258-263.

[23] Jiang Y, Zhao JJ, Mitlak BH, Wang O, Genant HK, Eriksen EF, 2003. Recombinant human parathyroid hormone (1-34) [teriparatide] improves both cortical and cancellous bone structure. *J. Bone Miner. Res.* 18, 1932-1941.

[24] Jilka RL, 2007. Molecular and cellular mechanisms of the anabolic effect of intermittent PTH. *Bone* 40, 1434-1446.

[25] JilkaRL, Weinstein RS, Bellido T, Roberson P, Parfitt AM, Manolagas SC, 1999. Increased bone formation by prevention of osteoblast apoptosis with parathyroid hormone. *J. Clin. Invest.* 104, 439-446.

[26] Kim HW, Jahng JS, 1999. Effect of intermittent administration of parathyroid hormone on fractures healing in ovariectomized rats. *Iowa Orthop. J.* 19, 71-77.

[27] Komatsubara S, Mori S, Mashiba T, Nonaka K, Seki A, Akiyama T, Miyamoto K, Cao Y, Manabe T, Norimatsu H, 2005. Human parathyroid hormone (1-34) accelerates the fracture healing process of woven to lamellar bone replacement and new cortical shell formation in rat femora. *Bone* 36, 678-687.

[28] Komrakova M, Stuermer EK, Werner C, Wicke M, Kolios L, Sehmisch S, Tezval M, Daub F, Martens T, Witzenhausen P, Dullin C and Stuermer KM 2010 Effect of human parathyroid hormone hPTH (1-34) applied at different regimes on fracture healing and muscle in ovariectomized and healthy rats. *Bone* 47, 480-492.

[29] Livak KJ, Schmittgen TD, 2001. Analysis of relative gene expression data using real-time quantitative PCR and the $2^{-\Delta\Delta CT}$ method. *Methods* 25, 402-408.

[30] Manabe T, Mori S, Mashiba T, Kaji Y, Iwata K, Komatsibara S, Seki A, Sun Y-X, Yamamoto T, 2007. Human parathyroid hormone (1-34) accelerates natural fracture healing process in the femoral osteotomy model of cynomolgus monkeys. *Bone* 40, 1475-1482.

[31] Namkung-Matthai H, Appleyard R, Jansen J, Hao Lin J, Maastricht S, Swain M, Mason RS, Murrell GA, Diwan AD, Diamond T, 2001. Osteoporosis influences the early period of fracture healing in a rat osteoporotic model. *Bone* 28, 80-86.

[32] Nakazawa T, Nakajima A, Shiomi K, Moriya H, Einhorn TA, Yamazaki M, 2005. Effects of low-dose, intermittent treatment with recombinant human parathyroid hormone (1-34) on chondrogenesis in a model of experimental fracture healing. *Bone* 37, 711-719.

[33] Nakajima A, Shimoji N, Shiomi K, Shimizu S, Moriya H, Einhorn TA, Yamazaki M, 2002. Mechanisms for the enhancement of fracture healing in rats treated with intermittent low-dose human parathyroid hormone (1-34). *J. Bone Miner Res.* 17, 2038-2047.

[34] Neer RM, Arnaud CD, Zanchetta JR, Prince R, Gaich GA, Reginster J-Y, Hodsman AB, Eriksen EF, Ish-Shalom S, Genant HK, Wang O, Mitlak BH. 2001. Effect of parathyroid hormone (1-34) on fractures and bone mineral density in postmenopausal women with osteoporosis. *N. Engl. J. Med.* 344, 1434-1441.

[35] Nozaka K, Miyakoshi N, Kasukawa Y, Maekawa S, Noguchi H, Shimada Y, 2008. Intermittent administration of human parathyroid hormone enhances bone formation and union at the site of cancellous bone osteotomy in normal and ovariectomized rats. *Bone* 42, 90-97.

[36] Rocca GJD, Crist BD, Murtha YM, 2010. Parathyroid hormone: is there a role in fracture healing. *J. Orthop. Trauma.* 24, S31-S35.

[37] Sehmisch S, Erren M, Rack T, Tezval M, Richter J, Seidlova-Wuttke D, Wuttke W, Stuermer KM, Stuermer EK, 2009. A new biomechanical test for intact rat lumbar vertebral bodies to study antiosteoporotic drugs. Short term effects of parathyroid hormone on rat lumbar vertebrae. *Spine* 34, 2014-2021.

[38] Shen V, Dempster DW, Mellish RWE, Birchman R, Horbert W, Lindsay R, 1992. Effects of combined and separate intermittent administration of low-dose human parathyroid hormone fragment (1-34) and 17β-estradiol on bone histomorphometry in ovariectomized rats with established osteopenia. Calcif Tissue Int. 50, 214-220.

[39] Stuermer EK, Sehmisch S, Rack T, Wenda E, Seidlova-Wuttke D, Tezval M, Wuttke W, Frosch KH and Stuermer KM, 2010. Estrogen and raloxifene improve metaphyseal fracture healing in the early phase of osteoporosis. A new fracture-healing model at the tibia in rat. *Langenbeck Arch. Surg*. 395, 163-172.

[40] Toro J, Tomin E, Shore B, Sull A, Morr S, Myers E, Lane JM, 2002. PTH and alendronate improve osteotomy healing in an osteoporotic rat model. *Eur. Cell Mater.* 13 (S2), 37.

[41] Wronski TJ, Yen C-F, 1994. Anabolic effects of parathyroid hormone on cortical bone in ovariectomized rats. *Bone* 15, 51-58.

[42] Yingjie H, Ge Z, Yisheng W, Ling Q, Hung WY, Kwoksui L, Fuxing P, 2007. Changes of microstructure and mineralized tissue in the middle and late phase of osteoporotic fracture healing in rats. *Bone* 41, 631-638.

Part 3:
Parathyroid Disorder

In: Parathyroid: Anatomy, Functions and Disorders
Editor: James Kirkby-Bott
ISBN: 978-1-62100-765-4

Chapter V

Familial Primary Hyperparathyroidism

***Radu Mihai*[1]**
John Radcliffe Hospital, Oxford
Nuffield Depart of Surgical Sciences, University of Oxford, UK

Abstract

Primary hyperparathyroidism is a common endocrine condition and in 1:10 patients it can occur as part of the recognised familial endocrine cancer syndromes - rare inherited autosomal dominant diseases with high penetrance. Identification of patients with familial PHPT is important for two main reasons. Firstly, the affected patients may be at risk from tumours that may arise in different glands, and regular screening for these tumours together with earlier treatment is expected to improve their prognosis. Secondly, the relatives of an affected patient are at a 50% risk of having inherited the mutation and thus developing such tumours.

These syndromes include multiple endocrine neoplasia type 1 (MEN1) and type 2 (MEN2), familial isolated primary hyperparathyroidism (FIHP), the hyperparathyroidism-jaw tumour syndrome (HPT-JT), familial benign hypocalciuric hypercalcaemia (FHH) and neonatal primary hyperparathyroidism (NHPT). Compared with sporadic PHPR, familial cases present at a younger age, are associated with multiglandular involvement and have a higher tendency to recur. The clinical features and their diagnosis, investigations and genetics, and management of each of these syndromes will be reviewed.

Introduction

Primary hyperparathyroidism (PHPT) is a very common endocrine condition with an annual incidence estimated to be approximately 20 per 100,000 and with a prevalence in postmenopausal women of 21 in 1000 population, which is equivalent to 3/1000 prevalence in the general population [1, 2]. Similarly, in a large cohort study in Scandinavia, the

[1]E-mail: radumihai@doctors.org.uk, Tel: +44 1865 221298, Fax: +44 1865 221189

prevalence of PHPT ranged from 0.5% in women 50-59 years old to 1.75% in women 70-75 years old [3]. Some 1:10 patients with PHPT develop the condition as part of a familial genetic trait and several autosomal dominant familial syndromes associated with PHPT have been described (Table 1). Compared with sporadic PHPT, familial cases present at a younger age, are more likely associated with multiglandular involvement and have a higher tendency to recur after surgical treatment.

Table 1. Familial endocrine cancer syndromes and their chromosomal locations

Disorder	OMIM Catalogue	Chromosomal location	Gene affected
MEN1	131100	11q13	MENIN
MEN2	171400	10q11.2	RET
FIHP	145000	1q25, 11q13	MENIN
HPT-JT	145001	1q31.2	PARAFIBROMIN
FHH, NHPT	145980 239200	3q21	CaSR

Details available from the Online Mendelian Inheritance in Man database (http://www.ncbi.nlm.nih.gov/omim).

Multiple Endocrine Neoplasia Type 1 (MEN1)

Multiple endocrine neoplasia (MEN) is characterised by the occurrence of tumours involving two or more endocrine glands within a single patient. The combined occurrence of tumours of the parathyroid glands, the pancreatic islet cells, and the anterior pituitary ("3Ps") is characteristic of multiple endocrine neoplasia type 1 (MEN1) whose eponim relates to Wermer's initial description of the first kindred [4]. It is estimated that only 12% of affected individuals manifest all three "P" lesions. In addition, endocrine tumours (adrenal cortical non-functional tumours, foregut carcinoids, thyroid neoplasms) and non-endocrine tumours (facial angiofibromas, collagenomas and lipomas, meningiomas, ependymomas) occur with variable penetrance.

MEN1 is an autosomal dominant disorder with an estimated incidence of 2-20/100,000 population [5]. It has a high degree of penetrance such that over 95% of affected individuals express signs of disease by the fifth decade. The earliest age at which manifestations of MEN1 may occur has been reported to be 5 years [6]. Lesions may develop multifocaly in the same gland, bilaterally in multiple glands at the same time (synchronous) or at variable intervals (metachronous) and tend to recur locally (if incompletely excised).

Genetics of MEN1. The gene causing MEN1 is localised on chromosome 11q13 and consists of 10 exons with a 1,830bp coding region that encodes a 610 amino acid protein, referred to as MENIN. Loss of heterozygosity involving chromosome 11q13 in affected individuals confirms the hypothesis that MEN1 gene acts as a tumour-suppressor gene, as expected from Knudson's model.

MENIN is ubiquitously expressed and has a variety of functions that include regulation of transcription, genome stability and cell division. In non-dividing cells *menin* is a nuclear protein while in dividing cells is found mainly in the cytoplasm. Truncated *menin* protein that would result from nonsense or frame-sift mutations lack the nuclear localisation signals. The majority of MEN1 mutations are likely to disrupt the interactions of menin with other proteins and thereby alter critical events in cell cycle regulation and proliferation [7]. Over 1300 mutations of MEN1 gene have been reported in the last decade [7]. The majority (70%) of these mutations are inactivating (truncating mutations, large deletions), consistent with those expected in a tumour suppressor gene. The mutations are scattered throughout the genomic sequence of the MEN1 gene with no evidence for clustering as observed in MEN2 (see below). A comparison of the clinical features in patients and their families with the same mutations reveals an absence of phenotype-genotype correlations. In addition, there is considerable variation in expression of the disease within families. This lack of genotype-phenotype correlations together with the wide diversity of mutations in the 1,830bp coding region of the MEN1 gene makes mutational analysis for diagnostic purposes in MEN1 time-consuming and expensive. Whilst genetic testing can identify patients some 20 years before the disease is clinically manifested, there is little benefit to be derived from such early diagnosis as it cannot predict the clinical pattern of future disease and prophylactic surgery is not feasible for parathyroid, pancreatic or pituitary tumours. A fascinating field is the ability to trace members of large families spanning many generations. For example the roots of eight Finish MEN1 families were raced back to a small village close to Oulu where the founder couple was born in early 1700 and whose offspring over 10 generations did not seem to have increased mortality [8]. In Brazil, three apparently unrelated genealogies came from a common Italian founder couple born in Venice in mid 1800 and who emigrated to Brazil in 1880 [9]. A subtype of MEN1 characterised to high incidence of prolactinoma (MEN1-Burin) was traced back to a small number of settlers who arrived from the southwest England in Newfoundland in early 1800s [10]. Similarly some 12 founder mutations were reported in MEN1 kindreds from Europe (France, Sweden), Oceania (Australia) and North America [11-13]. Clinical presentation of PHPT in MEN1 patients. PHPT is the most common feature of MEN1 as it occurs in 95% of all MEN1 patients. Furthermore PHPT is the presenting symptom in over two thirds of MEN1 patients. There is an equal male:female ratio (1M:1F) which contrasts with the female predominance in the sporadic PHPT (1M:3F). PHPT in MEN1 patients is unusual before the age of 15 years and the age of conversion from being unaffected to affected has been observed to be ≈20 years. Typically patients present in the third to fourth decade of life (i.e. earlier than sporadic PHPT), although significant variations exists among affected kindreds. Index patients may present with asymptomatic hyper-calcaemia or with vague symptoms associated with hypercalcaemia, for example polyuria, polydipsia, constipation and malaise. Occasionally patients present with nephrolithiasis and very rarely with osteitis fibrosa cystica or peptic ulcers. Bone mass in women with MEN1 is already low at 35 years of age [14, 15], presumably as a result of long-standing hyperpara-thyroidism and of a more severe impact on bone compared with patients with sporadic PHPT. Some reported that the first episode of urolithiasis occurs mostly before the age of 30 years [15], suggesting that kidney comorbidities may also begin at an early age. Biochemical parameters are usually mild and severe hypercalcaemia is a rare occurrence. Treatment of PHPT in MEN1 patients. There is no effective medical treatment for PHPT and surgical removal of the abnormal overactive parathyroid glands is the only definitive treatment. Several aspects related to parathyroidectomy in MEN1 patients continue to be debated:

1) Indications. It has been suggested that parathyroidectomy should be reserved for the symptomatic hypercalcaemic patient with MEN1, and that the asymptomatic hypercalcaemic MEN1 patient should not have parathyroid surgery but have regular assessments for the onset of symptoms and complications, when total parathyroidectomy should be undertaken.
2) Timing. Delayed procedures have the potential benefit of easier recognition of enlarged parathyroid glands. The concerns related to deferring surgical treatment is that in the absence of treatment, MEN1 parathyroid tumours result in significant morbidity in patients due to early-onset, frequent, extensive, severe and progressive bone and renal involvement (reviewed in [16]. There is therefore a tendency towards early parathyroidectomy in asymptomatic patients with mild hypercalcaemia, a strategy that has to acknowledge the increased the risk of recurrence and increasingly difficult reoperations.
3) The extent of parathyroid excision at the "ideal" first operation. All four parathyroid glands can be affected with multiple adenomas or hyperplasia but their enlargement is usually asymmetric and not all adenomas develop synchronously [17]. Bilateral neck exploration is the management of choice as it allows inspection of all four glands (Figure 1).
4) Less-than-subtotal parathyroidectomy has been abandoned in most centres because of its unacceptable high risk (35-60%) of persistent/recurrent disease. Subtotal parathyroidectomy (i.e. removal of all parathyroid glands leaving only a small remnant the size of 20-30 mg similar to a normal gland) is currently the most common procedure. In a study of 92 patients with MEN1 recurrence-free survival at 1, 5 and 10 years was 92%, 69% and 37% for patients who had 2.5 gland excision and 100%, 80% and 61% for those with more extensive resection [18]. In the largest series of MEN1-PHPT published to date, patients who underwent subtotal parathyroidectomy were 13-times more likely to have correction of hypercalcaemia compared with patients who lesser resection [19]. Furthermore, cumulative results in 544 patients from nine large series showed that within a 2-27 years follow-up some 15% of patients have either persistent disease or recurrent disease [20]. In a study from Uppsala, one of 15 patients who had total parathyroidectomy had persistent disease and only 20% had recurrent disease but 47% had severe postoperative hypocalcaemia [21]. Total parathyroidectomy with autotransplantation is favoured in some centres [22] and some report it to be equivalent to subtotal parathyroidectomy [23] but it is rarely considered for patients with MEN1.
5) The need for thymectomy. The rationale for thymectomy is that supranumerary glands and ectopic glands are common in MEN1 patient hence the cure of PHPT could be better if thymectomy is performed at the time of the initial neck exploration. Secondly, MEN1 patients are at risk of developing thymic carcinoids hence thymectomy might reduce the subsequent risk of developing such tumours. Though none of these facts have been challenged in randomised trials, it continues to be routine practice to perform thymectomy in MEN1 patients.

Diagnosis of index patients for MEN1 families. An aggressive policy of early screening is beneficial as those diagnosed by genetic-testing have less clinical manifestations when compared with those diagnosed clinically [24].

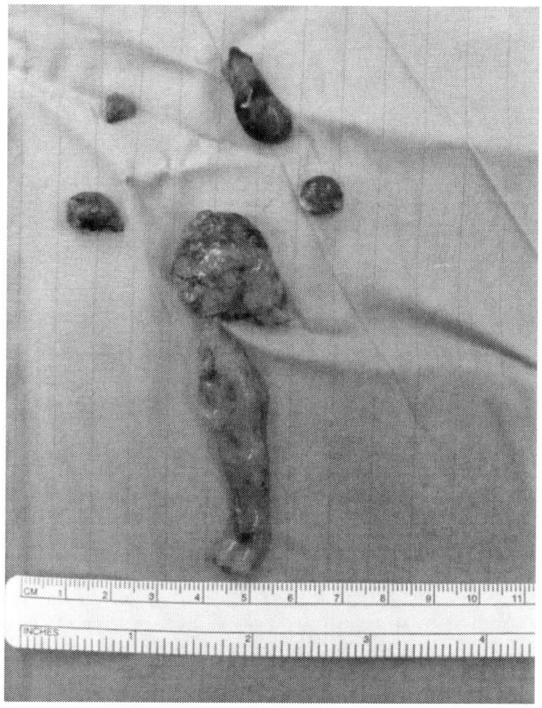

Figure 1. Extent of parathyroid involvement in a 31 yrs old man with MEN-1 primary hyperparathyroidism.

Screening for MEN-1 mutations in patients with PHPT is indicated in individuals with at least one of the following associated characteristics:

i)a first-degree relative with a major endocrine tumour

ii)parathyroid hyperplasia or associated multiple pancreatic tumours

iii)early age of onset. Prevalence of MEN-1 in patients 40 yrs with apparently sporadic PHPT is estimated at 13% [25]. In a report of 200 probands from Sweden the median age of those found to harbour a mutation was 33 yrs (range 9-71, n=49) compared with 50 yrs (range 7-86, n=150) in those without a mutations [26]. Based on such data international guidelines published in 2001 [27] recommend genetic screening of patients diagnosed with PHPT before 40 years of age. However, more recent publications showed there is no real basis for this management as several authors have reported that majority of patients 40 years have a single-gland disease and can be cured by limited parathyroidectomy, with only 5% of them having MEN1 gene mutations (Table 2), hence age alone should not be used as a criteria for instigating MEN1 screening.

Table 2. Incidence of MEN1 gene mutations in series of young patients with primary hyperparathyroidism

Ref	Selection criteria	Number of patients with hyperplasia	Number of patients with MEN1 gene mutations
USA, Mayo Clinic, [28]	<19 yrs	16%	
Finland, Oulu, [29]	<40 yrs		1/29
France, Marseille, [30]	<40 yrs		1/21
Germany, Neuss, [31]	<40 yrs	23% (vs 11% in patients >40 yrs)	
UK, Oxford (unpublished data)	<40 yrs		1/17
USA, Miami, [32]	<40 yrs	No difference between <40 and >40 yrs	
USA, Iowa, [33]	<40 yrs	no increased risk for MGD	
Japan, Kobe, [34]	1) <30 years old; 2) multigland disease; 3) associated MEN1-related tumors; 4) family history of PHPT or MEN1-related tumors.	15/60 (25%)	16/39 (41%)

Genetic screening of MEN-1 relatives. Screening of children of known MEN1 carriers should start early. Some consider at 5 years (as this is the earliest age reported) though in most series youngest patients are in their early teens.

Biochemical surveillance of mutation carriers. A prospective, nonrandomized study of 46 patients in a single German centre offering extensive clinical and biochemical annual screening program over a decade (1997-2006) found that the vast majority of lesions were nonprospectively diagnosed at initial evaluation. Though most patients are reviewed annually, the interval between screenings could be extended to 3 years based on annually calculated growth rates and the incidence of MEN-1-associated lesions. Biochemical screening (calcium, gastrin, and prolactin) should complement radiological screening (endoscopic ultrasound and CT/chest and abdomen)

Multiple Endocrine Neoplasia Type 2 (MEN2)

MEN2, which was initially referred to as *Sipple's syndrome*, describes the association of medullary thyroid carcinoma, phaeochromocytomas and parathyroid tumours. While medullary thyroid cancer develops in all gene carriers, phaeochromocytomas occur in half of patients and PHPT affects only 10%-30% of patients.

Genetics of MEN2. The gene causing MEN2 is located on chromosome 10cen-10q11.2. The *c-ret* proto-oncogene encodes a tyrosine kinase receptor with cadherin-like and cysteine-rich extracellular domains, and a tyrosine kinase intracellular domain. Specific mutations of *c-ret* have been identified for each of the three MEN2 variants. Thus in 95% of patients, MEN2a is associated with mutations of the cysteine-rich extracellular domain, and mutations in codon 634 (Cys→Arg) account for 85% of MEN2A mutations.

Most patients who develop PHPT have mutations in codon 634 [35], with variable penetrance between families who harbour this mutation. Since other codon mutations are rarely reported to lead to PHPT, there is no apparent genotype-phenotype correlation similar to the one reported for the onset of medullary thyroid carcinoma.

Clinical presentation of PHPT in MEN2 patients. Though some reported onset of the disease in patients as young as 9 years [36], most individuals are between second and fifth decade of life [37]. Majority of patients have minimal/no hypercalcaemia, and the presence of abnormally enlarged hyperplastic parathyroid(s) is usually revealed in the normocalcaemic patient undergoing thyroidectomy for MTC.

Operative strategy in MEN2. Before a neck operation patients should be screened biochemically for the presence of a phaeochromocytoma (if present, it should be operated before embarking on the neck operation). As parathyroidectomy is performed at the time of the thyroidectomy/central compartment dissection for MTC, great care should be taken to identify normal parathyroid glands and to avoid their devascularisation. If only one gland is enlarged, it should be the only one removed as limited parathyroidectomy in MEN2 leads to cure in some 90% of patients [38]. Others have questioned the role of limited parathyroidectomy as in their series there was only 77% cure rate of PHPT in MEN2, with 43% having ectopic glands and 8% having supranumerary glands [39] hence they suggest total parathyroidectomy with autotransplatation.

The advent of prophylactic thyroidectomy in children with RET mutations have brought the additional question of how to manage the parathyroid gland sin such children. As only 20-30% of MEN2 patients go on to develop PHPT, prophylactic parathyroidectomy has no role to play in this context. Normal glands should be identified and marked with a nonresorbable sutures and metal clips to facilitate future reoperations, if needed.

Hyperparathyroidism – Jaw Tumour (HPT-JT) Syndrome

The HPT-JT syndrome is a rare autosomal dominant disorder with incomplete penetrance and variable expression. As it was first described less than two decades ago [40], its real incidence is still unknown and arguably it is underestimated.

Genetics of HPT-JT. The *HRPT2* gene causing HPT-JT is located on chromosome 1q31.2. It encodes a 531 amino acid protein, *PARAFIBROMIN,* a ubiquitously expressed protein with antiproliferative properties. All reported mutations are predicted to result in a truncated or inactive parafibromin, in agreement with its tumour suppressor activity. In a recent review of 63 such families reported world-wide, some 67 of 245 affected individuals (27%) shown no clinical abnormalities [41] hence they can be described as *healthy mutation carriers.*

Loss of expression of parafibromin in all pathological tissue from HPT-JT-related tumours is a distinguishing feature of the syndrome. Parafibromin immunostaining should therefore be used as a screening test for all pathological tissue suspected to be related to HPT-JT before embarking on the more expensive (and sparsely available) genetic tests.

Clinical presentation of PHPT in HPT-JT syndrome. Hyperparathyroidism is the most common feature but with incomplete penetrance (~70%). As a general trend, parathyroid tumours occur at an earlier age (youngest reported patient was 11 yrs old, majority of patients are in their 30s). Some 90% of affected individuals have single-gland disease and the rest have synchronous multigland-involvement. There is a high prevalence of parathyroid carcinomas (~27%, though the figures might represent reporting bias) and atypical adenomas.

PHPT is associated with non-endocrine tumours which define the syndrome:

- associated ossifying fibromas of mandible and/or maxilla are the distinguishing feature of HPT-JT and may occasionally precede the development of hypercalcaemia in HPT-JT patients by several decades. The jaw tumours in HPT-JT are different to the brown tumours observed in some patients with sporadic PHPT and do not resolve after parathyroidectomy. It is important to emphasise that these abnormalities were observed in only a quarter of 245 patients from 63 families (Iacobone, Masi et al. 2009) hence in the absence of a personal or family history of jaw tumours the condition might be misdiagnosed.
- uterine tumours derivative of Mullerian duct system occur in two thirds of patients (leyomiomas, endometrial hyperplasia, adenomyosis, adenofibromas, adeno-sarcoma).
- various renal lesions (renal cysts, Wilms' tumours, renal hamartomas, renal cortical adenomas, papillary renal cell carcinomas) may develop in some 16% of patients
- pancreatic adenocarcinomas, testicular mixed germ cell tumours with a major seminoma component, and Hurthle cell thyroid adenomas have been occasionally reported.

It is important to note that the parathyroid tumours may occur in isolation and without any evidence of jaw tumours, and this may cause confusion with other hereditary hypercalcaemic disorders such as MEN1 and familial benign hypercalcaemia (FHH, see below). HPT-JT can be distinguished from FBH, as in FBH the serum calcium is elevated from the early neonatal or infantile period, whereas in HPT-JT such elevations are uncommon in the first decade. In addition, HPT-JT unlike FBH patients will have associated hypercalciuria.

The distinction between HPT-JT patients and MEN1 patients, who have only developed the usual first manifestation of hypercalcaemia (90% of patients), is more difficult and is likely to be influenced by the operative and histological findings and the occurrence of other characteristic lesions in each disorder. It is important to note that HPT-JT patients will usually have single adenomas or a carcinoma, whilst MEN1 patients will often have multiglandular and hyperplastic parathyroid disease. These distinctions may be helped by the identification of additional features, and a search for jaw tumours, renal, pancreatic, thyroid and testicular abnormalities may help to identify HPT-JT patients.

In more recent case series reported after identification of HRPT2 gene mutations an increasing number of patients have single-gland disease (~90%), low recurrence rate (~22%) and (relatively) low risk of parathyroid carcinomas. It is reasonable therefore that limited parathyroidectomy (i.e. scan-directed minimally invasive parathyroidectomy when feasible) is considered optimal treatment.

Furthemore, recurrence occurs after a long interval (mean 14 yrs) due to further single gland enlargement and cure at reoperation can be achieved by selective parathyroidectomy [41]. Others have suggested extensive parathyroidectomy as in MEN-1 patients but this strategy appears excessive for HPT-JT patients.

Familial Hypocalciuric Hypercalcaemia and Neonatal Primary Hyperparathyroidism

Familial hypocalciuric hypercalcaemia (FHH), which is also referred as familial benign hypercalcaemia, is an autosomal dominant disorder with a high degree of penetrance that is characterised by lifelong asymptomatic hypercalcaemia in association with an inappropriately low urinary calcium excretion (calcium clearance to creatinine clearance ratio 0.01).

A normal circulating PTH concentration and mild hypermagnesaemia are also typically present. Although most patients with FHH are asymptomatic, chondrocalcinosis and acute pancreatitis have occasionally been observed to occur in some patients.

In addition, children of consanguineous marriages within FHH kindreds have been observed to have life-threatening hypercalcaemia due to neonatal primary hyperparathyroidism (NHPT). NHPT is defined as symptomatic hypercalcaemia with skeletal manifestations of hyperparathyroidism in the first 6 months of life [42]. NHPT children often present in the first few days or weeks of life with failure to thrive, dehydration, hypotonia, constipation, rib cage deformities and multiple fractures due to bony undermineralisation. Children with NHPT often require urgent parathyroidectomy, which corrects the PTH-dependent hypercalcaemia and bone demineralisation.

Genetics. FHH is due to heterozygous inactivating mutations of the calcium sensing receptor (CaSR) and NHPT is often associated with inactivating homozygous CaSR mutations. However, NHPT has also been observed in children where only one parent had clinically apparent FHH, and many other NHPT patients appear to be sporadic, i.e. with both parents being normocalcaemic. In such NHPT patients with heterozygous CaSR mutations, the mutant CaSR may exert a dominant negative action on the normal CaSR. The human CaSR is a 1078 amino-acid cell surface protein which is expressed in parathyroids, thyroid cells and kidney, and is a member of the family of G-protein coupled receptors [42]. The CaSR gene is located on chromosome 3q21.1. In addition to the loss of function CaSR mutations which result in FHH and NHPT, gain of function CaSR mutations resulting in autosomal dominant hypocalcaemia with hypercalciuria have also been reported [42]

The clinical importance of FHH lies in its differentiation from primary hyperparathyroidism (see above) as patients with FHH should not be offered parathyroid surgery. The diagnosis of FHH should be considered when hypercalcaemia is diagnosed in young patients who might have a family history of hypercalcaemia and failed parathyroid surgery and who are found to have low 24-hours urine excretion (1.5-2 mmol/24h). The diagnosis is confirmed by demonstrating a low (1%) urinary calcium clearance to creatinine clearance ratio, which is calculated based on the formula CaCl/CrCl = Cau × Crs / Cas × Cru.

Familial Isolated Primary Hyperparathyroidism (FIHP)

Hereditary PHPT may develop as a solitary endocrinopathy, and this has also been referred to as familial isolated HPT (FIHP). Over 100 families with FIHP have been reported [43, 44]. FIHP is characterized by earlier onset, higher incidence of multiglandular disease, and higher recurrence rate when compared with sporadic primary hyperparathyroidism

Genetics of FIHP. This is a heterogeneous group of conditions with abnormalities reported in the following genes:

- MEN-1 gene [43]. 41% of these are missense mutations and 37% are frame-shift or nonsense mutations that are predicted to result in a truncated protein [43]. This contrast significantly with the situation in MEN1 syndrome, in whom less than 20% of the germline mutations are missense and more than 80% are protein-truncating [7]
- CaSR gene- 5 kindreds [45]
- putative gene on chromosome 2p13-14 – 9 kindreds [46]

Cases of FIHPT should be offered a thorough genetic screening to avoid confusion with other known syndromes with incomplete penetrance (MEN1, HPT-JT) and to guide the long-term follow-up surveillance for the development of other tumours.

As the genetic basis of this syndrome varies between families the aggressiveness of surgical strategy (i.e. limited or subtotal parathyroidectomy) has to be adapted to each kindred.

Subtotal parathyroidectomy (excision of 3½ or 4 glands with autotransplantation) has been recommended [47]. The downside if this approach is a risk of permanent hypoparathyroidism in 13% to 41% of patients.

It has been reported that many patients with FIHPT return to normocalcaemia after single-gland excision. In one such study, 15 consecutive patients with FIHPT underwent limited parathyroidectomy with resection guided by intact parathyroid hormone secretion. With an operative success of 93%, 14 patients had only single-gland excision and 80% had unilateral neck exploration. All initial patients had their hypercalcaemia corrected. In 4 reoperations, permanent hypoparathyroidism occurred in 2 patients. One recurrence was observed in 40 (8-122) months of follow-up [48].

Conclusion

- Familial endocrine disease is uncommon.
- Multigland hyperplasia is the commonest presenting phenotype in MEN 1 and causes more severe hypercalcaemia than in MEN 2 disease.
- HPT-JT syndrome is linked to parathyroid carcinoma via parafibromin expression
- Familial isolated hyperparathyroidism is a multigland phenomena associated via a variety of mutations.

References

[1] Heath, H., 3rd, S.F. Hodgson, and M.A. Kennedy, Primary hyperparathyroidism. Incidence, morbidity, and potential economic impact in a community. *N. Engl. J. Med*, 1980. 302(4): p. 189-93.

[2] Adami, S., C. Marcocci, and D. Gatti, Epidemiology of primary hyperparathyroidism in Europe. *J. Bone Miner. Res*, 2002. 17 Suppl 2: p. N18-23.

[3] Jorde, R., K.H. Bonaa, and J. Sundsfjord, Primary hyperparathyroidism detected in a health screening. The Tromso study. *J. Clin. Epidemiol*, 2000. 53(11): p. 1164-9.

[4] Wermer, P., Endocrine Adenomatosis and Peptic Ulcer in a Large Kindred. Inherited Multiple Tumors and Mosaic Pleiotropism in Man. *Am. J. Med*, 1963. 35: p. 205-12.

[5] Carling, T., Multiple endocrine neoplasia syndrome: genetic basis for clinical management. *Curr. Opin. Oncol*, 2005. 17(1): p. 7-12.

[6] Stratakis, C.A. and D.W. Ball, A concise genetic and clinical guide to multiple endocrine neoplasias and related syndromes. *J. Pediatr. Endocrinol. Metab*, 2000. 13(5): p. 457-65.

[7] Lemos, M.C. and R.V. Thakker, Multiple endocrine neoplasia type 1 (MEN1): analysis of 1336 mutations reported in the first decade following identification of the gene. *Hum. Mutat*, 2008. 29(1): p. 22-32.

[8] Ebeling, T., et al., Effect of multiple endocrine neoplasia type 1 (MEN1) gene mutations on premature mortality in familial MEN1 syndrome with founder mutations. *J. Clin. Endocrinol. Metab*, 2004. 89(7): p. 3392-6.

[9] Lourenco, D.M., Jr., et al., Multiple endocrine neoplasia type 1 in Brazil: MEN1 founding mutation, clinical features, and bone mineral density profile. *Eur. J. Endocrinol*, 2008. 159(3): p. 259-74.

[10] Olufemi, S.E., et al., Common ancestral mutation in the MEN1 gene is likely responsible for the prolactinoma variant of MEN1 (MEN1Burin) in four kindreds from Newfoundland. *Hum. Mutat*, 1998. 11(4): p. 264-9.

[11] Vasen, H.F., C.B. Lamers, and C.J. Lips, Screening for the multiple endocrine neoplasia syndrome type I. A study of 11 kindreds in The Netherlands. *Arch. Intern. Med*, 1989. 149(12): p. 2717-22.

[12] Toledo, R.A., et al., Novel MEN1 germline mutations in Brazilian families with multiple endocrine neoplasia type 1. *Clin. Endocrinol.* (Oxf), 2007. 67(3): p. 377-84.

[13] Vierimaa, O., et al., Multiple endocrine neoplasia type 1 in Northern Finland; clinical features and genotype phenotype correlation. *Eur. J. Endocrinol*, 2007. 157(3): p. 285-94.

[14] Burgess, J.R., et al., Osteoporosis in multiple endocrine neoplasia type 1: severity, clinical significance, relationship to primary hyperparathyroidism, and response to parathyroidectomy. *Arch. Surg*, 1999. 134(10): p. 1119-23.

[15] Lourenco, D.M., Jr., et al., Early-onset, progressive, frequent, extensive, and severe bone mineral and renal complications in multiple endocrine neoplasia type 1-associated primary hyperparathyroidism. *J. Bone Miner. Res*. 25(11): p. 2382-91.

[16] Brandi, M.L., Parathyroid gland: Hyperparathyroidism in MEN1 syndrome: time to operate? *Nat. Rev. Endocrinol*, 2010. 6(11): p. 604-5.

[17] Doherty, G.M., T.C. Lairmore, and M.K. DeBenedetti, Multiple endocrine neoplasia type 1 parathyroid adenoma development over time. *World J. Surg*, 2004. 28(11): p. 1139-42.

[18] Elaraj, D.M., et al., Results of initial operation for hyperparathyroidism in patients with multiple endocrine neoplasia type 1. *Surgery*, 2003. 134(6): p. 858-64; discussion 864-5.

[19] Goudet, P., et al., Hyperparathyroidism in multiple endocrine neoplasia type I: surgical trends and results of a 256-patient series from Groupe D'etude des Neoplasies Endocriniennes Multiples Study Group. *World J. Surg*, 2001. 25(7): p. 886-90.

[20] Stalberg, P. and T. Carling, Familial parathyroid tumors: diagnosis and management. *World J. Surg*, 2009. 33(11): p. 2234-43.

[21] Hellman, P., et al., Primary and reoperative parathyroid operations in hyperparathyroidism of multiple endocrine neoplasia type 1. *Surgery*, 1998. 124(6): p. 993-9.

[22] Tonelli, F., et al., Is total parathyroidectomy the treatment of choice for hyperparathyroidism in multiple endocrine neoplasia type 1? *Ann. Surg*, 2007. 246(6): p. 1075-82.

[23] Waldmann, J., et al., Surgery for multiple endocrine neoplasia type 1-associated primary hyperparathyroidism. *Br. J. Surg*, 2010. 97(10): p. 1528-34.

[24] Pieterman, C.R., et al., Multiple endocrine neoplasia type 1 (MEN1): its manifestations and effect of genetic screening on clinical outcome. *Clin. Endocrinol.* (Oxf), 2009. 70(4): p. 575-81.

[25] Langer, P., et al., Prevalence of multiple endocrine neoplasia type 1 in young patients with apparently sporadic primary hyperparathyroidism or pancreaticoduodenal endocrine tumours. *Br. J. Surg*, 2003. 90(12): p. 1599-603.

[26] Tham, E., et al., Clinical testing for mutations in the MEN1 gene in Sweden: a report on 200 unrelated cases. *J. Clin. Endocrinol. Metab*, 2007. 92(9): p. 3389-95.

[27] Brandi, M.L., et al., Guidelines for diagnosis and therapy of MEN type 1 and type 2. *J. Clin. Endocrinol. Metab*, 2001. 86(12): p. 5658-71.

[28] Kollars, J., et al., Primary hyperparathyroidism in pediatric patients. *Pediatrics*, 2005. 115(4): p. 974-80.

[29] Vierimaa, O., et al., Mutation analysis of MEN1, HRPT2, CASR, CDKN1B, and AIP genes in primary hyperparathyroidism patients with features of genetic predisposition. *J. Endocrinol. Invest*, 2009. 32(6): p. 512-8.

[30] Skandarajah, A., et al., Should routine analysis of the MEN1 gene be performed in all patients with primary hyperparathyroidism under 40 years of age? *World J. Surg*, 2007. 34(6): p. 1294-8.

[31] Wirowski, D., et al., Does multiple gland disease in primary hyperparathyroidism correlate with age or sex? *Langenbecks Arch. Surg*, 2009. 394(5): p. 885-90.

[32] Sneider, M.S., et al., Sporadic primary hyperparathyroidism in young individuals: different disease and treatment? *J. Surg. Res*, 2009. 155(1): p. 100-3.

[33] Adam, L.A., et al., Role for limited neck exploration in young adults with apparently sporadic primary hyperparathyroidism. *World J. Surg*, 2008. 32(7): p. 1518-24.

[34] Kihara, M., et al., MEN1 gene analysis in patients with primary hyperparathyroidism: 10-year experience of a single institution for thyroid and parathyroid care in Japan. *Endocr. J*, 2009. 56(5): p. 649-56.

[35] Schuffenecker, I., et al., Risk and penetrance of primary hyperparathyroidism in multiple endocrine neoplasia type 2A families with mutations at codon 634 of the RET proto-oncogene. Groupe D'etude des Tumeurs a Calcitonine. *J. Clin. Endocrinol. Metab*, 1998. 83(2): p. 487-91.

[36] Jackson, M.B., et al., Multiple endocrine neoplasia type 2A in a kindred with C634Y mutation. *Pediatrics*, 2005. 116(3): p. e468-71.

[37] Yip, L., et al., Multiple endocrine neoplasia type 2: evaluation of the genotype-phenotype relationship. *Arch. Surg*, 2003. 138(4): p. 409-16; discussion 416.

[38] Raue, F., et al., Primary hyperparathyroidism in multiple endocrine neoplasia type 2A. *J. Intern Med*, 1995. 238(4): p. 369-73.

[39] Herfarth, K.K., et al., Surgical management of hyperparathyroidism in patients with multiple endocrine neoplasia type 2A. *Surgery*, 1996. 120(6): p. 966-73; discussion 973-4.

[40] Jackson, C.E., et al., Hereditary hyperparathyroidism and multiple ossifying jaw fibromas: a clinically and genetically distinct syndrome. *Surgery*, 1990. 108(6): p. 1006-12; discussion 1012-3.

[41] Iacobone, M., et al., Hyperparathyroidism-jaw tumor syndrome: a report of three large kindred. *Langenbecks Arch. Surg*, 2009. 394(5): p. 817-25.

[42] Thakker, R.V., Genetics of endocrine and metabolic disorders: parathyroid. *Rev. Endocr. Metab. Disord*, 2004. 5(1): p. 37-51.

[43] Pannett, A.A., et al., Multiple endocrine neoplasia type 1 (MEN1) germline mutations in familial isolated primary hyperparathyroidism. *Clin. Endocrinol.* (Oxf), 2003. 58(5): p. 639-46.

[44] Simonds, W.F., et al., Familial isolated hyperparathyroidism: clinical and genetic characteristics of 36 kindreds. *Medicine* (Baltimore), 2002. 81(1): p. 1-26.

[45] Carling, T., et al., Familial hypercalcemia and hypercalciuria caused by a novel mutation in the cytoplasmic tail of the calcium receptor. *J. Clin. Endocrinol. Metab*, 2000. 85(5): p. 2042-7.

[46] Warner, J.V., et al., Familial isolated hyperparathyroidism is linked to a 1.7 Mb region on chromosome 2p13.3-14. *J. Med. Genet*, 2006. 43(3): p. e12.

[47] Hannan, F.M., et al., Familial isolated primary hyperparathyroidism caused by mutations of the MEN1 gene. *Nat. Clin. Pract. Endocrinol. Metab*, 2008. 4(1): p. 53-8.

[48] Carneiro, D.M., G.L. Irvin, 3rd, and W.B. Inabnet, Limited versus radical parathyroidectomy in familial isolated primary hyperparathyroidism. *Surgery*, 2002. 132(6): p. 1050-4; discussion 1055.

In: Parathyroid: Anatomy, Functions and Disorders
Editor: James Kirkby-Bott
ISBN: 978-1-62100-765-4

Chapter VI

Parathyroid Disorders in Children and Adolescents

Pisit Pitukcheewanont and Rudruidee Karnchanasorn
[1]Center of Endocrinology, Diabetes and Metabolism, Children's Hospital Los Angeles, Department of Pediatrics, The Keck School of Medicine of University of Southern California, Los Angeles, California, US
[2]Department of Clinical Diabetes, Endocrinology, and Metabolism, City of Hope National Medical Center, Duarte, California, US

Abstract

Childhood parathyroid disorders are rare phenomena. Primary, Secondary and Tertiary hyperparathyroidism can occur in children and adolescents in a similar manner as to in adults, though in primary HPT they are more likely to have a familial syndrome. Neonatal and childhood hypoparathyroid occurs due to: inherited genetic syndromes, gland damage during neck surgery, copper deposition or exposure to ionising radiation. Preterm infants are at risk of a transient hypoparathyroid hypocalcaemia. Children can present with acute symptoms such as tetany, cardiac conduction abnormalities and GI upset. Autoimmune causes can be associated with adrenal insufficiency which needs to be looked for in the assessment of these patients.

Introduction

Parathyroid disorders in children and adolescents are not uncommon. In this chapter we will discuss the etiologies, evaluations and treatment of hypoparathyroidism, pseudohypoparathyroidism and primary hyperparathyroidism in children and adolescents.

Hypoparathyroidism

Hypoparathyroidism results from defective synthesis, secretion, or action of parathyroid hormone (PTH), end-organ resistance, or inappropriate regulations that result from the activated or antibody-stimulated calcium-sensing receptor (CaSR) [1]. These defects can be inherited or acquired. PTH secretion by the parathyroid glands (prime regulators of serum calcium concentration) maintains serum calcium within a strict range. Biochemical hallmarks of hypoparathyroidism include hypocalcemia and hyperphosphatemia, in the setting of normal or inappropriately low PTH level. Pseudohypoparathyroidism (PHP) is diagnosed when patients presented with hypoparathyroidism but the PTH levels are elevated. The incident of hypoparathyroidism and PHP in the United States has not been reported. In Japan, a recent survey found the prevalence of idiopathic hypoparathyroidism to be 7.2 cases per million people and the prevalence of PHP to be 3.4 cases per million people [2].

Parathyroid Physiology

Mature PTH is an 84–amino acid peptide. Production and secretion of PTH are regulated by a G protein–coupled calcium-sensing receptor. Unlike other protein hormones, its production and secretion are stimulated by decreased intracellular calcium concentrations, which reflect by low serum calcium concentrations. PTH exerts its action through the PTH receptor, which is another member of the G protein–linked receptor family. The type 1 PTH receptor found in bones, kidneys, and intestines are essential in calcium and phosphate homeostasis. The type 2 PTH receptor has been found in the brain and intestines which binds to a different peptide and its function is not known [3].

The net effects of PTH activity are an increase in serum calcium and a decrease in serum phosphate. PTH acts directly on bone to stimulate bone resorption and cause calcium and phosphate release. PTH acts directly on the kidney to decrease calcium clearance and to inhibit phosphate reabsorption. By stimulating renal 1-alpha-hydroxylase activity, PTH increases serum concentrations of 1, 25-dihydroxyvitamin D, the active form of vitamin D and, thus, indirectly stimulates calcium and phosphate absorption by the gut through the actions of vitamin D. The phosphaturic effect of PTH offsets the increases of serum phosphate driven by increased bone resorption and GI absorption.

Hypoparathyroidism results in loss of the direct and indirect effects of PTH on bone, the kidney, and the gut. Calcium and phosphate release from bone is impaired, calcium absorption from the gut is limited, calciuria develops despite hypocalcemia, and retention of phosphate from the urine causes increased plasma phosphate levels.

Causes

Hypoparathyroidism may be transient, genetically inherited, or acquired. Genetically inherited forms arise from defects of parathyroid gland development, defects in the parathyroid hormone (PTH) gene, defects in the calcium-sensing receptor gene, defects in

PTH action, defects in the autoimmune regulator gene, and genetic syndromes. Acquired hypoparathyroidism may be due to an autoimmune process or may occur after neck irradiation or surgery.

- Transient hypoparathyroidism occurs during the neonatal period. Preterm infants are at increased risk, and as many as 50% of very low birth weight infants may have a deficient surge in PTH that results in hypocalcemia. Hypocalcemia is noted in 10-20% of infants of diabetic mothers. These infants may be born prematurely, which is a risk factor for insufficient PTH response. They may have hypomagnesemia from maternal magnesuria complicating glucosuria which impairs PTH release and action [4]. PTH secretion is suppressed in the fetus because of high placental transfer of calcium, particularly in the third trimester. With cord clamping, calcium transfer abruptly stops; serum calcium concentrations decrease rapidly, and PTH secretion is triggered. Prolonged delay in PTH responsiveness in some otherwise healthy infants causes transient hypoparathyroidism. Maternal hypercalcemia from hyperparathyroidism can also cause prolonged suppression of PTH secretion in the neonate.
- DiGeorge syndrome and velocardiofacial syndrome are associated with abnormal development of the third and fourth pharyngeal pouches from which the parathyroids derive embryologically and represents an example of a defect in parathyroid gland development. DiGeorge syndrome and velocardiofacial syndrome are variants of the chromosome arm 22q11 microdeletion syndrome. They occur in approximately 1:4000 births [5]. Several cases of chromosome 10p deletion have also been reported in which affected individuals have some features of DiGeorge syndrome. Hypocalcemia associated with a 22q11 microdeletion may be transiently present in infancy but recur later in life, particularly during periods of stress. Hypocalcemia can be the only manifestation of this disorder. Patients with chromosome arm 22q11.2 microdeletion who present with late-onset hypoparathyroidism in adolescence have been described [5-6].
- X-linked recessive hypoparathyroidism has been associated with parathyroid agenesis and has been mapped to chromosome arm Xq26-q27, the location of a putative developmental gene [7].
- Familial cases of hypoparathyroidism due to mutations of the PTH gene located on chromosome arm 11p15 have been identified. These mutations have been both dominantly and recessively inherited [8].
- Autosomal recessive forms of hypoparathyroidism have been shown to be caused by rare homozygous mutations in the genes encoding pre-pro-PTH or glial cell missing B (GCMB) [9].
- Autosomal dominant forms of hypoparathyroidism could be due to a dominant negative GCMB mutation [10].
- Polyendocrinopathy-candidiasis-ectodermal dystrophy syndrome, also known as APS I, has been linked to loss-of-fuction mutations of an autoimmune regulator gene located on chromosome band 21q22.3 [11]. Patients with hypoparathyroidism of APS I usually present within the first few years of life after the onset of chronic mucocutaneous candidiasis and before the onset of adrenal insufficiency. More than 75% of individuals with APS I develop hypoparathyroidism, more than 85% of patients develop adrenal insufficiency, and 60% of women have ovarian failure. Due

to wide spectrum of clinical manifestations of APS I, a lifelong monitoring for the development of new components of APS I is indicated [12].

- The hypoparathyroidism, deafness, and renal dysplasia (HDR) syndrome is an autosomal dominant disorder associated with partial monosomy of chromosome arm 10p.
- Mitochondrial cytopathies, such as Kearns-Sayre syndrome (ie, external ophthalmoplegia, ataxia, sensorineural deafness, heart block, and elevated cerebral spinal fluid (CSF) protein), are associated with Hypoparathyroidism [13].
- Hypoparathyroidism-retardation-dysmorphism (HRD) syndrome and Kenny-Caffey syndrome have also been associated with hypoparathyroidism. Mutations in the *TBCE* gene, which encodes a chaperone protein required for alpha tubulin subunit folding, have been identified in both disorders [14].
- Hypoparathyroidism incurred during neck surgery may be transient or permanent depending upon the extent of injury and preservation of the parathyroid glands. Rates following surgical procedures such as thyroidectomy vary depending on the extent of the surgery and experience of the surgeon. Transient hypoparathyroidism occurs in approximately 10% of the patients undergoing total thyroidectomy. Less than half of these patients develop permanent hypoparathyroidism (hypoparathyroidism that persists longer than 6 months after surgery) [15]. Parathyroid autotransplantation can be used to preserve parathyroid function, however with high failure late and risk for late auto graft-medicated recurrences of hyperparathyroidism [3].
- Hypoparathyroidism following months after radioactive iodine ablation of the thyroid has been described as more common in treatment of Grave disease than with treatment of thyroid cancer. Radiation to the chest or neck area for cancer is also associated with hypoparathyroidism.
- Parathyroid gland destruction due to deposition of iron (as with hemochromatosis or multiple blood transfusions) or deposition of copper (as with Wilson disease) has been described [16-17].
- Calcium-sensing receptor (CaSR) mutations represent a resetting of the calciostat and are not considered an etiology of a true hypoparathyroid state. However, patients present with hypocalcemia, inappropriate normal PTH levels, and mild-to-moderate elevations of phosphate levels, and, hence, mimic hypoparathyroidism. Patients may present with hypocalcemia any time from birth to adulthood. Autosomal dominant and sporadic gain-of-function mutations of the Ca^{2+} receptor, a G-protein coupled receptor, cause hypocalcemic hypercalciuria by lowering the serum calcium concentration that is required for PTH secretion and urinary calcium reabsorption [18-19]. Individuals with Ca^{2+} receptor mutations have PTH concentrations that are within the reference range in the setting of hypocalcemia; they can be asymptomatic or severely affected. These individuals must be differentiated from individuals with true hypoparathyroidism because treatment with active vitamin D (calcitriol) can cause nephrocalcinosis and renal insufficiency by exacerbating the already high urinary calcium excretion. Therapy with calcitriol should be restricted to symptomatic individuals and should be sufficient enough to relieve symptoms without normalizing serum calcium concentrations.

- Treatment with thiazide diuretics has been shown to be beneficial. In addition, PTH therapy could be effective in correcting serum and urine calcium and the phosphate levels in this disorder [20].

Presentation

Clinical Manifestations of hypoparathyroidism result from hypocalcemia. Severe hypocalcemia presents with seizures, stridor, prolonged QTc, refractory heart failure, and tetany, especially when it occurs acutely. Patient with chronic hypoparathyroidism can be asymptomatic or may develop cataract, ectopic calcification (basal ganglia), and occasionally parkinsonism and dementia.

Complications of hypocalcemia:

- Neurologic: Neuromuscular irritability, peri - oral or acral paresthesia, carpopedal spasm, muscle twitching, tetany, or seizures. Neck muscle cramping can cause dystonic like neck movements.
- Cardiac: Prolongation of the QTc interval, arrhythmia, or heart failure. Affected individuals may be asymptomatic or experience syncope, seizure, or death due to arrhythmias, such as polymorphic ventricular tachycardia.
- Respiratory: Laryngospasm and bronchospasm can lead to stridor and significant airway obstruction.

History

Review of the past medical history or symptoms are very helpful in determining the etiology of the hypoparathyroidism.

- DiGeorge syndrome and velocardiofacial syndrome are associated with recurrent infections related to T-cell abnormalities and conotruncal cardiac abnormalities, such as tetralogy of Fallot and truncus arteriosus. Affected individuals may also have a history of speech delay from velopharyngeal insufficiency [5].
- Familial autoimmune polyglandular syndrome type I (APS I) is associated with chronic mucocutaneous candidiasis, adrenal insufficiency, and hypoparathyroidism. (Two of these conditions are required for diagnosis)[3]. It could be associated with type 1 diabetes mellitus, hypogonadism, or hypothyroidism. Other nonendocrine manifestations of this autoimmune syndrome include vitiligo, pernicious anemia, dental enamel hypoplasia, and malabsorbtion. Candidal infections of the skin or GI tract that last more than 3 months are considered chronic and are the presenting symptom in 60% of individuals with hypoparathyroidism due to APS I.
- A history of radioactive iodine ablation of the thyroid for Grave disease may predate the development of acquired hypoparathyroidism by several months. However, it could be sooner in those patients who underwent thyroid surgery.
- Sensorineural deafness, renal dysplasia, and mental retardation are also associated with syndromes of hypoparathyroidism, deafness, and renal anomalies.

Physical Examination

- Hyperreflexia due to hypocalcemia is common.
- Trousseau sign is a carpopedal spasm that occurs after a blood pressure cuff around the arm is inflated above the systolic blood pressure for several minutes.
- Chevstok sign (twitching of ipsilateral facial muscles with tapping on the facial nerve in front of the ear and just below the zygomatic bone) is a manifestation of neuromuscular excitability. Chevstok sign is present in 25% of healthy adults and in even higher rates in children. Thus, its presence or absence should be documented prior to thyroidectomy.
- Chromosome band 22q11 deletion/velocardiofacial syndrome/DiGeorge syndrome has characteristic physical features, but hypoparathyroidism may be the only immediately recognizable manifestation.
- Nasal speech can occur from a cleft palate or velopharyngeal insufficiency.
- Bulbous nasal tip, micrognathia, ear anomalies, and short philtrum are typical facial features but may not be evident in nonwhite children.
- A heart murmur may signify a conotruncal heart defect.
- Short stature may be a feature of the genetic syndrome, but in some cases, it is due to growth hormone deficiency.

Laboratory Data

- Total and ionized serum calcium: In hypoparathyroidism, total and ionized calcium levels are low. Ionized calcium level should be evaluated in patients with hypoalbuminemia.
- Serum phosphate: Serum phosphate levels are elevated, although they can be within the reference range, especially in the infant without enteral feeding and low phosphate/protein intake.
- Serum magnesium: Serum magnesium levels are obtained to rule out hypomagnesemia as a cause of hypoparathyroidism. In this condition, hypocalcemia could be corrected very rapidly with magnesium therapy. In general, magnesium levels are within the reference range in hypoparathyroidism.
- Intact parathyroid hormone (iPTH): Obtain iPTH at the time of hypocalcemia. Nomograms have been developed for the interpretation of serum iPTH concentration with respect to the serum calcium. In hypoparathyroidism, iPTH is low. An iPTH that falls within the reference range must be interpreted with caution. The value might be considered low in the face of hypocalcemia..
- BUN and creatinine levels: BUN and creatinine concentrations are obtained to assess renal function. These test results are normal in hypoparathyroidism
- 25-hydroxyvitamin D and 1,25-dihydroxyvitamin D: 25-Hydroxyvitamin D and 1,25-dihydroxyvitamin D concentrations are obtained to rule out a vitamin D–deficient or vitamin D–resistant state as the etiology of hypocalcemia. 25-Hydroxyvitamin D levels are within the reference range in hypoparathyroidism. 1,25-Dihydroxyvitamin D levels are expected to be low in hypoparathyroid states because

of lack of PTH-stimulated 1-alpha-hydroxylase activity. Urine calcium and creatinine ratio: Urine calcium is elevated in PTH-resistant and PTH-deficient states and particularly elevated in calcium-sensing receptor mutations.

- Thyroid studies comprising: Thyroid-stimulating hormone [TSH], thyroxine, and thyroid antibodies [antiperoxidase and antithyroglobulin antibodies]. If an autoimmune process is suspected as the etiology of hypoparathyroidism, thyroid studies may uncover a concomitant hypothyroid state. TSH resistance can be associated with PHP Ia.
- Adrenocorticotropic hormone (ACTH) and adrenal antibodies: If an autoimmune process is suspected, concomitant primary adrenal insufficiency can be revealed by an elevated ACTH level, and adrenal antibodies may be present.

Radiological Studies

- Chest radiography: Thymic aplasia is associated with the 22q11 deletion syndrome and can be assessed with chest radiography.
- Echocardiography: An infant with a murmur and in whom hypoparathyroidism is suggested should have echocardiography performed to assess for conotruncal lesions that are associated with the 22q11 deletion syndrome.
- Renal ultrasonography: Treatment of hypoparathyroidism can lead to nephrocalcinosis as a result of hypercalciuria. Baseline renal ultrasonography with initial treatment should be performed.
- Brain MRI: Basal ganglia calcifications are commonly presented in hypoparathyroidism. These suggest a long-standing presence of calcium disorder. These calcifications can occur even before the treatment of hypocalcemia was initiated.

Other Tests

- Electrocardiography: A prolonged QTc interval is found with hypocalcemia and resolves with correction of serum calcium.
- ACTH stimulation testing: Adrenal insufficiency can be life threatening. If APS I is suggested, an ACTH stimulation study should be performed to assess adrenal function (if basal ACTH levels are elevated).
- Thyrotropin-releasing hormone stimulation testing: PHP Ia is associated with generalized hormone resistance. Hypothyroidism may be subtle and may only be detected with a thyrotropin-releasing hormone (TRH) stimulation study. Unfortunately, TRH is not commercially available at this time.
- Genetic studies, when applicable.
- In neonates, a fluorescence in situ hybridization (FISH) for the chromosome band 22q11 deletion.

Management

Symptomatic hypocalcemia (eg, seizure, tetany, laryngospasm) in patients with hypoparathyroidism requires intravenous calcium and continuous monitoring for cardiac arrhythmias.

Oral calcium and active vitamin D (calcitriol) should be initiated as soon as possible (eg, when the patient is tolerating oral feeds). Once serum calcium concentrations are in a safe range (7.5 mg/dL), intravenous calcium can be stopped.

Prolonged intravenous calcium therapy with existing high serum phosphate will increase further precipitation of calcium-phosphate compound. However, rebound hypocalcemia can occur and requires that a patient be monitored for therapeutic success on oral agents for at least 24 hours after intravenous calcium is withdrawn. In patients with hungry bone syndrome, prolonged intravenous calcium therapy may be needed.

The active form of vitamin D, 1,25-dihydroxyvitamin D (calcitriol), is preferred in the treatment of hypoparathyroidism because both the parathyroid hormone (PTH) deficiency/resistance and the hyperphosphatemia impair the activation of 25-hydroxyvitamin D by 1-alpha-hydroxylase.

Pseudohypoparathyroidism (PHP)

Pseudohypoparathyroidism results from targeted organ (kidney and bone) unresponsiveness to PTH. Resistance to PTH is characterized by hypocalcemia, hyper-phosphatemia and elevated PTH concentrations. This syndrome has been divided in to PHP type 1 and PHP type 2.

Pseudohypoparathyroidism Type 1 is caused by mutation of the GNAS1 gene. The GNAS1 gene encodes the alpha subunit of the G protein, coupled to the PTH receptor that mediates cyclic AMP stimulation by PTH and other peptide hormones including thyrotropin. GNAS1 is imprinted, therefore the expression of the allele for a specific tissue is dependent on whether the allele is maternally or paternally inherited [21]. The patients with PHP type 1 have diminished urinary cyclic AMP response to exogenous PTH administration.

Pseudohypoparathyroidism Type 1a or Albright's hereditary osteodystrophy (AHO) is inherited as an autosomal dominant trait and associated with other skeletal abnormality and additional hormone resistance. Individuals with PHP type 1a have the typical features characteristics of AHO.

They are obese, have short stature and short fourth and fifth metacarpals/metatarsals, and may have subcutaneous calcifications and disturbances of taste, smell, hearing, and vision. Patients also have mental retardation and developmental delay. Maternal transmission of the mutation is required for expression of this syndrome [22].

Pseudo-pseudohypoparathyroidism (PPHP) is inherited from the paternal allele of a mutated GNAS1 gene and presents with Albright osteodystrophy without evidence of hypoparathyroidism due to normal renal responsiveness to PTH from the normal maternal allele [23].

Pseudohypoparathyroidism Type 1b presents with hypoparathyroidism without the AHO phenotype [24]. The mutated allele is maternally transmitted.

Table 6.1. Clinical features and abnormal genes in pseudohypoparathyrodism and pseudopseudohypoparathyroidism

Type	AHO	GSα	GNAS1 gene
PHP Ia	+	↓	Paternal imprinting
PHP Ib	-	WNL	Paternal imprinting
PHP Ic	-	WNL	?
PHP II	-	WNL	Post-receptor defect
PPHP	+	↓	Maternal imprinting

PHP: Pseudohypoparathyroidism, PPHP: Pseudopseudohypoparathyroidism WNL : Within Normal Limits AHO: Albright's hereditary osteodystrophy Gsα: GNAS gene, G protein coupling receptor.

Pseudohypoparathyroidism Type 1c has the same manifestation as PHP type 1a but it is caused by mutations that affect the coupling of the G protein to the PTH receptor [25].

Pseudohypoparathyroidism Type2 affected individuals have no clinical features of AHO and have normal or elevated urinary cyclic AMP concentrations in response to exogenous PTH administration but without a concomitant increase in phosphate excretion [26]. The mutation defect of this syndrome has not been reported.

Laboratory and Radiological Studies

Individuals with PHP present with low serum calcium and elevated serum phosphate with elevated iPTH. Serum magnesium, renal function, serum 25-OH vitaminD are usually normal. Elevated 1,25-dihydroxyvitamin D concentrations have been documented in PHP, but the mechanism remains unclear. Left hand and wrist radiography (bone age) show brachymetacarpals (shortening of fourth and fifth metacarpals) that are a feature of Albright hereditary osteodystrophy (AHO) phenotype and can aid in the diagnosis of PHP Ia. There may be some degrees of advanced bone age in those patients with PHP. Basal ganglia calcifications from brain MRI are also present in PHP, and found more commonly than hypoparathyroidism. Table 2 outlines biochemical and clinical parameters that can help distinguish sub-types of PHP from PPHP.

Table 6.2. Clinical and Laboratory Findings in Patients with Pseudohypoparathyroidism and Pseudopseudohypoparathyroidism

	Calcium	Phosphate	iPTH	Urinary cAMP	Urine Pi	TSH	AHO	Gsα Activity	GSα Mutation
PHPIa	↓	↑	↑	↓	↓	(↑)	+	↓	+
PHPIb	↓	↑	↑	↓	→	→	-	→	-(?)
PHP Ic	↓	↑	↑	↓	-	(↑)	+	-	-
PHPII	↓	↑	↑	→	↓	→	-	→	-(?)
PPHP	→	→	→	→	→	→	+	↓	+

PHP: Pseudohypoparathyroidism, PPHP: Pseudopseudohypoparathyroidism.
AHO: Albright's hereditary osteodystrophy.
Pi: inorganic phosphate, Urine cAMP and urine Pi : the response after PTH administration.

Management

The treatment of hypocalcemia in patients with pseudohypoparathyroidism type 1a or 1b are similar to patients with true hypoparathyroidism.

Primary Hyperparathyroidism in Children

Primary hyperparathyroidism (PHPT) is a rare condition in Children and is uncommon in adolescents [27]. The incidence of PHPT is approximately 2-5 in 100,000 and it mostly occurs in adolescents (74%-88%) [28]. Previous reports suggested equal distribution or slight male predominance, but a recent study showed a higher female-to-male ratio of 7:2[29], compared to 6:5 [30] and 3:2 [28] in other series. PHPT is most commonly caused by a parathyroid adenoma but it may be associated with multiple endocrine neoplasia (MEN) type1 or 2 syndrome, or familial non-MEN hyperparathyroidism [28]. The genetic defect in sporadic parathyroid adenoma is linked to cyclin D1 or PRAD1 overexpression [31]. Parathyroid hyperplasia is uncommon in children in compared to adults [30] and it is more often expressed as familial forms of hyperparathyroidism. MEN1 is transmitted in autosomal dominant fashion and related with menin gene defect located at chromosome 11q13[32]. PHPT is often the first manifestation. In contrast, PHPT occurs less commonly in MEN type 2A and is rarely the first manifestation of this syndrome. MEN type2A is associated with the RET proto oncogene defect in chromosome 10q11.2 in autosomal dominant fashion [33]. Parathyroid carcinoma is also rare in children and can be related to retinoblastoma tumor suppressor gene[34]. Neonatal severe primary hyperparathyroidism is a rare and lethal disease associated with homozygous inactivating germ-line mutations of the calcium-sensing receptor gene. Patients have an enlargement of all parathyroid glands and very elevated serum calcium [3]. The diagnosis of PHPT is often delayed because of non specific presenting symptoms, therefore the majority of patients present with end organ damage [28, 30].

History and Physical Examination

Previous reports suggest that symptoms in children with PHPT are more severe than adults. In a large cohort of 52 children and adolescents, 79% children were symptomatic at presentation. The most common presenting symptoms are fatigue and lethargy (35%), headache (35%), nephrolithiasis (33%), nausea (29%), abdominal pain (25%), vomiting (23%), and polydipsia (21%). Skeletal abnormalities in patients with primary hyperparathyroidism include bone pain, muscle weakness, brown tumors and rarely rickets. Physical examination in a patient with PHPT is mostly unremarkable; only a few patients present with a palpable parathyroid mass [28].

PHPT may cause end-organ damage involvement to the eyes, kidneys, and skeletal system. 33% of patients who had a slit lamp examination performed in one series developed band keratopathy [30]. 44% of Patients from the Mayo clinic developed kidney damage, including nephrocalcinosis (8%), nephrolithiasis (33%), and bone involvement (34%). Bone involvement was more common in younger patients. Acute pancreatitis is also reported (7%) [28]. The prevalence of end-organ damage has decreased recently with the increased use of serum calcium level in routine paediatric assessment [30].

Laboratory and Radiology Studies

PHPT usually presents with hypercalcemia, low to normal serum phosphate, and inappropriately high PTH levels. However, normocalcemic primary hyperparathyroidism has been reported to occur in patients with vitamin D deficiency [35]. A report from India, where suboptimal vitamin D supplementation was widely prevalent, indicated that serum calcium levels were within normal range in almost half of patients with primary hyperparathyroidism at the initial presentation [36], reflecting the opposing effects of excess PTH secretion and vitamin D deficiency on calcium levels. Serum alkaline phosphatase level in children is more variable than adults, making this test less reliable. Hypercalciuria is common but to the lesser extent than other non-parathyroid causes of hypercalcemia. Unless urinary calcium is low which suggests familial hypocalciuric hypercalcemia, urinary calcium excretion is less helpful in children [30]. However it is important to correct vitamin D in patients with a normal calcium and elevated PTH as the PTH may normalise with vitamin D replacement and PHPT is not present in such patients.

Abnormal radiological findings include osteitis fibrosa cystica, subperiosteal bone resorption and pathological fractures [28, 30, 36]. However, among the radiological abnormalities, rickets is rarely reported. Only sixteen patients presenting with rickets as the presenting manifestation of PHPT have been reported in the English literature and there is only one patient reported as presenting with vitamin D deficient rickets due to an ectopic thymic parathyroid adenoma [35]. Vitamin D deficiency has been shown to be associated with severe skeletal damage in patients with primary hyperparathyroidism, as previously reported in developing countries such as India [36] and among Asian immigrants in Britain [37]. Lower intake of vitamin D and calcium in India than in the United States was considered to be responsible for the persistence of large parathyroid tumors and osteitis fibrosa cystica in affected patients [38]. Recent studies demonstrated that the effects of primary hyperparathyroidism on biochemical, densitometric, and histomorphometric indices of skeletal metabolism were more pronounced in patients with a low 25(OH)D [39-40].

Radiologic studies used in preoperative localization have included ultrasonography, magnetic resonance imaging, computed tomography, nuclear scans, and selective angiography. Ultrasonography is the most commonly used study in paediatric patients with a sensitivity of 86%, specificity of 67%, and a positive predictive value of 95% [28].

The sensitivity of each study modality has improved over the years with the reported sensitivity as high as 100% for nuclear scans and 80% for ultrasound and CT since year 2000 in children [29]. Ectopic parathyroid glands are more common in children with higher failure rate of primary operation, 20% compared to 2% in adults; therefore greater attention to preoperative localization is recommended [28].

Management

Parathyroidectomy is the main treatment of hyperparathyroidism in children and adolescents. Operative treatment consists of cervical exploration with single-gland parathyroidectomy for isolated adenoma and subtotal parathyroidectomy or total parathyroidectomy with autotransplantation for multiple-gland disease or hyperplasia such as MEN or familial hyperplasia [28]. Post-operative complications include permanent and transient hypocalcemia and vocal cord injury. Hungry bone syndrome presenting with severe hypocalcemia, hypophosphatemia, tetany, peri-oral tingling and numbness was reported in 27.7% of patients from a paediatric study in India [29]. Long-term complications such as permanent hypocalcemia, hypercalcemia, and permanent recurrent laryngeal nerve injury are uncommon . The success rate for operative treatment in pediatric patients is excellent. Medical management of PHPT are available with the calcimimetic, cinacalcet, which is an allosteric modulator of the calcium-sensing receptor (CaSR). Cinacalcet increases the sensitivity of CaSR to the extracellular Ca concentration and reduces PTH release[42]. Cinacalcet has been approved by the U.S. food and drugs Administration for treatment of secondary hyperparathyroidism (SHPT) in patients with chronic kidney disease on dialysis and for treatment of parathyroid carcinoma. Although it is not currently approved for the treatment of PHPT, it reduces serum calcium and PTH levels in patients with mild PHPT [43-45] and also PHPT patients across a wide spectrum of disease severity[46]. Cinacalcet was approved by the European commission for the treatment of hypercalcemia in patients with PHPT for whom parathyroidectomy is contraindicated. There is no improvement of bone mineral density with cinacalcet compared to placebo [44] but it should be consider in patients with PHPT whom are not candidates for surgery[47].

Secondary and Tertiary Hyperparathyroidism

Secondary parathyroid hyperplasia (SHPT) results from elevated levels of PTH in response to low serum calcium or 1,25 vitamin D due to various conditions. These include chronic kidney diseases, renal tubular acidosis, intestinal malabsorption, inadequate vitamin D and calcium intake, treatment of hypophosphatemic rickets, cholestatic liver disease, and iatrogenic causes such as lithium. Patients with SHPT normally present with their underlying disease. Serum calcium increases gradually to a higher set point for PTH suppression that eventually can lead to tertiary hyperparathyroidism (THPT) when PTH secretion becomes insuppressible [48]. This occurs after long standing end stage renal failure and is discussed in the chapter on renal HPT. Laboratory and Radiologic Studies.

In SHPT, serum calcium is low or normal with elevated PTH levels, in contrast to elevation of both serum calcium and phosphorus in PHPT. Serum phosphorus is elevated in patients with SHPT due to chronic renal failure. In THPT, PTH level are persistently elevated, although serum calcium and phosphorus are normalized.

Abnormal radiological findings are useful in defining the level of severity in SHPT. Cortical bone is primarily affected, as opposed to cancellous or trabecular bone.

Management

Cinacalcet has been reported to be successful in treatment of SHPT in children. Calcitriol is used for patients with SHPT due to end stage renal failure. Parathyroidectomy is indicated when medical management fails or when THPT develops.

Conclusion

Biochemical hallmarks of hypoparathyroidism are hypocalcemia and hyperphosphatemia. Pseudohypoparathyroidism is characterized by hypocalcemia, hyperphosphatemia and elevated PTH concentrations. Severe hypocalcemia presents with seizures, stridor, prolonged QTc, refractory heart failure, and tetany. Treatment of symptomatic hypocalcemia requires intravenous calcium, while calcium and 1,25-dihydroxyvitamin D are the main treatment of chronic hypocalcemia secondary to hypoparathyroidism.

PHPT is uncommon in children but associated with significant morbidity. Suspected children should be screened by checking serum calcium and PTH. Normocalcemic primary hyperparathyroidism may occur in patients with vitamin D deficiency. Preoperative localization with ultrasound and/or nuclear scan is recommended. Parathyroidectomy is effective and is a treatment of choice in children with PHPT, however, cinacalcet is the promising therapy especially when surgery is contraindicated.

Secondary Hyperparathyroidism is resulted from elevated level of PTH in response to low serum calcium or elevated serum phosphate due to various underlying diseases especially chronic renal failure, malabsorption and inadequate calcium and vitamin D intake. Cinacalcet is approved for treatment of secondary hyperparathyroidism in patients with chronic kidney disease on dialysis and for treatment of parathyroid carcinoma. Parathyroidectomy is indicated when medical management fails or when THPT developed.

References

[1] Roth KS, W.R., Chan JCM, Sarafoglou K. , *Disorders of calcium, phosphate, and bone metabolism*. Pediatric endocrinology and inborn errors of metabolism.ed. Vol. 2009. 2009, New York, NY: McGraw Hill.

[2] Nakamura, Y., et al., *Prevalence of idiopathic hypoparathyroidism and pseudohypoparathyroidism in Japan. J. Epidemiol*, 2000. 10(1): p. 29-33.

[3] Marx, S.J., *Hyperparathyroid and hypoparathyroid disorders. N. Engl. J. Med*, 2000. 343(25): p. 1863-75.

[4] Shoback, D., *Clinical practice. Hypoparathyroidism. N. Engl. J. Med*, 2008. 359(4): p. 391-403.

[5] McDonald-McGinn, D.M. and K.E. Sullivan, *Chromosome 22q11.2 Deletion Syndrome (DiGeorge Syndrome/Velocardiofacial Syndrome). Medicine* (Baltimore), 2011. 90(1): p. 1-18.

[6] Cuneo, B.F., *22q11.2 deletion syndrome: DiGeorge, velocardiofacial, and conotruncal anomaly face syndromes. Curr. Opin. Pediatr*, 2001. 13(5): p. 465-72.

[7] Trump, D., et al., *Localisation of X linked recessive idiopathic hypoparathyroidism to a 1.5 Mb region on Xq26-q27. J. Med. Genet*, 1998. 35(11): p. 905-9.

[8] Tsukamoto, K. and M. Emi, *A polymorphic CA repeat sequence at the human calcitonin locus. J. Hum. Genet*, 1998. 43(2): p. 146-7.

[9] Baumber, L., et al., *Identification of a novel mutation disrupting the DNA binding activity of GCM2 in autosomal recessive familial isolated hypoparathyroidism. J. Med. Genet*, 2005. 42(5): p. 443-8.

[10] Mannstadt, M., et al., *Dominant-negative GCMB mutations cause an autosomal dominant form of hypoparathyroidism. J. Clin. Endocrinol. Metab*, 2008. 93(9): p. 3568-76.

[11] Aaltonen, J., et al., *An autosomal locus causing autoimmune disease: autoimmune polyglandular disease type I assigned to chromosome 21. Nat. Genet*, 1994. 8(1): p. 83-7.

[12] Eisenbarth, G.S. and P.A. Gottlieb, *Autoimmune polyendocrine syndromes. N. Engl. J. Med*, 2004. 350(20): p. 2068-79.

[13] Zahirieh, A., et al., *Functional analysis of a novel GATA3 mutation in a family with the hypoparathyroidism, deafness, and renal dysplasia syndrome. J. Clin. Endocrinol. Metab*, 2005. 90(4): p. 2445-50.

[14] Parvari, R., et al., *The 2p21 deletion syndrome: characterization of the transcription content. Genomics*, 2005. 86(2): p. 195-211.

[15] Khan, M.I., S.G. Waguespack, and M.I. Hu, *Medical Management of Postsurgical Hypoparathyroidism. Endocr. Pract*, 2010: p. 1-19.

[16] Angelopoulos, N.G., et al., *Hypoparathyroidism in transfusion-dependent patients with beta-thalassemia. J. Bone Miner. Metab*, 2006. 24(2): p. 138-45.

[17] Carpenter, T.O., D.L. Carnes, Jr., and C.S. Anast, *Hypoparathyroidism in Wilson's disease. N. Engl. J. Med*, 1983. 309(15): p. 873-7.

[18] Brown, E.M., *Clinical lessons from the calcium-sensing receptor. Nat. Clin. Pract. Endocrinol. Metab*, 2007. 3(2): p. 122-33.

[19] Pollak, M.R., et al., *Autosomal dominant hypocalcaemia caused by a Ca(2+)-sensing receptor gene mutation. Nat. Genet*, 1994. 8(3): p. 303-7.

[20] Shiohara, M., et al., *Effect of parathyroid hormone administration in a patient with severe hypoparathyroidism caused by gain-of-function mutation of calcium-sensing receptor. Endocr. J*, 2006. 53(6): p. 797-802.

[21] Bastepe, M. and H. Juppner, *GNAS locus and pseudohypoparathyroidism. Horm. Res*, 2005. 63(2): p. 65-74.

[22] Nakamoto, J.M., et al., *Pseudohypoparathyroidism type Ia from maternal but not paternal transmission of a Gsalpha gene mutation. Am. J. Med. Genet*, 1998. 77(4): p. 261-7.

[23] Davies, S.J. and H.E. Hughes, *Imprinting in Albright's hereditary osteodystrophy. J. Med. Genet*, 1993. 30(2): p. 101-3.

[24] Liu, J., et al., *A GNAS1 imprinting defect in pseudohypoparathyroidism type IB. J. Clin. Invest*, 2000. 106(9): p. 1167-74.

[25] Farfel, Z., et al., *Pseudohypoparathyroidism: inheritance of deficient receptor-cyclase coupling activity. Proc. Natl. Acad. Sci. U S A*, 1981. 78(5): p. 3098-102.

[26] Rodriguez, H.J., et al., *Pseudohypoparathyroidism type II: restoration of normal renal responsiveness to parathyroid hormone by calcium administration. J. Clin. Endocrinol. Metab*, 1974. 39(4): p. 693-701.

[27] Allo, M., et al., *Primary hyperparathyroidism in children, adolescents, and young adults. World J. Surg*, 1982. 6(6): p. 771-6.

[28] Kollars, J., et al., *Primary hyperparathyroidism in pediatric patients. Pediatrics*, 2005. 115(4): p. 974-80.

[29] George, J., et al., *Primary hyperparathyroidism in children and adolescents. Indian. J. Pediatr*, 2010. 77(2): p. 175-8.

[30] Lawson, M.L., et al., *Primary hyperparathyroidism in a paediatric hospital. QJM*, 1996. 89(12): p. 921-32.

[31] Arnold, A., et al., *Molecular pathogenesis of primary hyperparathyroidism. J. Bone Miner. Res*, 2002. 17 Suppl 2: p. N30-6.

[32] Mayr, B., et al., *Menin mutations in patients with multiple endocrine neoplasia type 1. Eur. J. Endocrinol*, 1997. 137(6): p. 684-7.

[33] Eng, C. and L.M. Mulligan, *Mutations of the RET proto-oncogene in the multiple endocrine neoplasia type 2 syndromes, related sporadic tumours, and hirschsprung disease. Hum. Mutat*, 1997. 9(2): p. 97-109.

[34] Cryns, V.L., et al., *Loss of the retinoblastoma tumor-suppressor gene in parathyroid carcinoma. N. Engl. J. Med*, 1994. 330(11): p. 757-61.

[35] Pitukcheewanont, P., N. Numbenjapon, and G. Costin, *Ectopic thymic parathyroid adenoma and vitamin D deficiency rickets: a 5-year-follow-up case report and review of literature. Bone*, 2008. 42(4): p. 819-24.

[36] Harinarayan, C.V., N. Gupta, and N. Kochupillai, *Vitamin D status in primary hyperparathyroidism in India. Clin. Endocrinol.* (Oxf), 1995. 43(3): p. 351-8.

[37] Sultan, A.H., F.E. Bruckner, and J.B. Eastwood, *Association between prolonged dietary vitamin D deficiency and autonomous hyperparathyroidism. BMJ*, 1989. 299(6693): p. 236-7.

[38] D.S. Rao, E.P., M. Honasoge, A. Mithal, S.C. Mishra and A.K. Sing et al., *Role of vitamin D nutrition in primary hyperparathyroidism: effect on parathyroid gland mass and on bone.* Vitamin D: chemistry, biology, and clinical applications of the steroid hormone, ed. R.B.a.M.T. A.W. Norman. 1997, Riverside, California.

[39] Vieth, R., *Vitamin D supplementation, 25-hydroxyvitamin D concentrations, and safety. Am. J. Clin. Nutr*, 1999. 69(5): p. 842-56.

[40] Wharton, B. and N. Bishop, *Rickets. Lancet*, 2003. 362(9393): p. 1389-400.

[41] Udelsman, R., *Surgery in primary hyperparathyroidism: the patient without previous neck surgery. J. Bone Miner. Res*, 2002. 17 Suppl 2: p. N126-32.

[42] Rao, L.G. and M.S. Kung, *Effect of long-term and short-term diabetes on the parathyroid hormone sensitive rat renal adenylate cyclase: correlation with vitamin D metabolism. Can. J. Physiol. Pharmacol*, 1988. 66(10): p. 1313-8.

[43] Marcocci, C., et al., *Cinacalcet reduces serum calcium concentrations in patients with intractable primary hyperparathyroidism. J. Clin. Endocrinol. Metab*, 2009. 94(8): p. 2766-72.

[44] Peacock, M., et al., *Cinacalcet hydrochloride maintains long-term normocalcemia in patients with primary hyperparathyroidism. J. Clin. Endocrinol. Metab*, 2005. 90(1): p. 135-41.

[45] Shoback, D.M., et al., *The calcimimetic cinacalcet normalizes serum calcium in subjects with primary hyperparathyroidism. J. Clin. Endocrinol. Metab*, 2003. 88(12): p. 5644-9.
[46] Peacock, M., et al., *Cinacalcet HCl reduces hypercalcemia in primary hyperparathyroidism across a wide spectrum of disease severity. J. Clin. Endocrinol. Metab*, 2011. 96(1): p. E9-18.
[47] Khan, A., A. Grey, and D. Shoback, *Medical management of asymptomatic primary hyperparathyroidism: proceedings of the third international workshop. J. Clin. Endocrinol. Metab*, 2009. 94(2): p. 373-81.
[48] Rivkees, S.A., et al., *Tertiary hyperparathyroidism during high phosphate therapy of familial hypophosphatemic rickets. J. Clin. Endocrinol. Metab*, 1992. 75(6): p. 1514-8.

In: Parathyroid: Anatomy, Functions and Disorders
Editor: James Kirkby-Bott

ISBN: 978-1-62100-765-4

Chapter VII

Parathyroid Carcinoma

Filomena Cetani and Claudio Marcocci[2]
Department of Endocrinology and Metabolism, University of Pisa, Pisa Italy

Abstract

Parathyroid carcinoma (PC) accounts for less than 1% of cases of sporadic primary hyperparathyroidism (PHPT) and is usually associated with more severe clinical manifestations than parathyroid adenoma. Its course is typically indolent, but progressive. The diagnosis of malignancy is often made only when local recurrence or metastases occur, because the histology of parathyroid tumors can be equivocal or frankly misleading. Surgery is the only curative treatment for PC and consists of complete resection of the primary lesion at the time of initial operation. For this reason, both preoperative suspicion and intraoperative recognition are of great importance. Despite a potentially curative resection, PC has a recurrence rate of more than 50%. Most recurrences occur 2-3 years after the initial operation, but this period is variable and a prolonged disease-free interval of as long as 20 years has been reported. Most patients with recurrent disease ultimately succumb to the effects of hypercalcemia, rather than to direct tumor invasion or distant metastases. Recently, the calcimimetic cinacalcet, an allosteric modulator of the calcium sensing receptor, has be effectively employed to control hypercalcemia in patients with metastatic disease in whom surgical options were exhausted.

Introduction

Parathyroid carcinoma (PC) is a rare cause of primary hyperparathyroidism (PHPT) [1]. It accounts for less than 1% of cases of sporadic PHPT and is usually associated with more severe clinical manifestations than its much more common benign counterpart, parathyroid adenoma. PC has a rather indolent course [2-4]. The definite diagnosis can be made at histology but in most cases is made in retrospect when local recurrence or metastases occur,

[2]Department of Endocrinology and Metabolism, University of Pisa, Via Paradisa 2 56124 Pisa, Italy

because in some cases the histology can be equivocal or frankly misleading [4, 5]. The prognosis of PC is quite variable, but most patients die because of severe hypercalcemia due to hyper-secretion of PTH by metastatic tissues. A successful resection of the tumor at initial surgery is the main determinant of the prognosis. Clinical clues to the possibility of a PC, therefore, should lead the surgeon to an aggressive initial operative approach. In the last decade, greater knowledge of the molecular pathogenesis of PC has led to the development of diagnostic markers that show promise, particularly when the histology is ambiguous [4,-6]. Moreover, there is the hope that the understanding of the carcinogenesis process will led to the development of new therapeutic strategies for advanced, inoperable disease.

Epidemiology

Approximately 400 case of PC have been reported [7]. Most of them are sporadic but familial cases have also been described. The largest series of 286 cases has been collected by the National Cancer Database [8]. In most series of PHPT, PC accounts for less than 1% of cases, but an incidence as high as 5% has been reported [3, 9, 10]; the use of different histological criteria likely accounts for this discrepancy.

At variance with its benign counterpart, the incidence of PC is matched between the sexes. The age at diagnosis is 10 yr earlier than the typical age when the benign form of PHPT presents (mid-40s vs. mid-50s).

Aetiology

The etiology of PC is unknown. Prior neck irradiation is a risk factor of PHPT [11-15], but the role of radiation in PC is not clear. PC has been described rarely in patients with longstanding secondary hyperparathyroidism due to chronic end-stage renal failure [16, 17] and in one patient with celiac disease [17]. In the few such cases, it is unclear whether the currently accepted pathological criteria of parathyroid malignancy were met. PC has also been reported in association with hereditary hyperparathyroidism syndromes [18-21]. It occurs in 15% of patients with the hyperparathyroidism-jaw tumor (HPT-JT) syndrome [22]. HPT-JT is a rare autosomal dominant disorder where hyperparathyroidism is due to a neoplasm of one or more parathyroid glands. In HPT-JT, cystic changes in the parathyroid tumors are common, and this disorder has also been referred to as cystic parathyroid adenomatosis [23]. Ossifying fibromas of the maxilla and mandible are found in 30% of patients. Less commonly, kidney lesions, including cysts, polycystic disease, hamartomas, or Wilm's tumors can be present [24]. PC has also been reported in association with familial isolated hyperparathyroidism [19,20, 25]. A few recent reports have suggested that PC, as defined pathologically, may occur in a setting of MEN1 syndrome and/or tumors carrying somatic *MEN1* mutations [26-29]. However, recurrent parathyroid disease in MEN1 may mimic, but not actually be due to malignancy. Only one case of PC has been reported in the MEN2A syndrome [30]. .

Molecular Pathogenesis

Oncogenes and tumor suppressor genes and/or their products, especially those involved in the control of the cell cycle [retinoblastoma (Rb), p53, breast carcinoma susceptibility (BRCA2), Ki-67 and cyclin Dl/parathyroid adenomatosis gene 1 oncogene (PRAD1)], have been linked to PC [31-39] (Table 7.1). Early studies provided promising results on the use of markers as diagnostic tool of PC, but further investigations showed an overlap between benign and malignant lesions [33-39]. Recent studies of exon 3 of the *CTNNB1* gene encoding ®-catenin showed absence of stabilizing mutations in PC [40]. In addition losses or gains in various chromosomal loci have been identified in PCs, suggesting that genes located in these chromosomes might be involved in aberrant parathyroid growth [32]. The HPT-JT syndrome has provided the best evidence for a defined gene in PC. The gene is known now as *HRPT2* but other terms have been used, such as *CDC73* and *Clorf* 28 [24]. Several evidences indicate a strong association between *HRPT2* mutations and PC [41-43]. *HRPT2* is the target for germline mutation in the majority of families with the rare HPT-JT, in which PC occurs at higher frequency than in sporadic PHPT series (15% vs. 1%). Similar germline mutations occur in a subset of kindreds with familial isolated hyperparathyroidism [24, 41-50]. The role of the *HRPT2* gene in the pathogenesis of sporadic PC was first demonstrated by Howell and co-workers [41] who detected *HRPT2* mutations in four of four PC and in none of 25_sporadic parathyroid adenomas. Subsequently, Shattuck et al. [42] found *HRPT2* mutations in 10 of 15 patients with apparently sporadic PC. Cetani et al. identified *HRPT2* mutations in 9 out of 11 PC and in none of 4 sporadic atypical adenomas [43]. Most of the mutations are nonsense and predicted to result in lack of or reduced protein expression of the encoded parafibromin protein (see below). Combining the results of these studies, the prevalence of *HRPT2* mutations in sporadic PCs was 76.6 %. Inactivating *HRPT2* mutation in non-coding or regulatory regions could be implicated in cases without alterations in the coding regions of the gene. Of particular interest is the demonstration that germline *HRPT2* mutations were identified in one third of patients [28, 42, 43, 51]. This finding suggests that a subset of patients with apparently sporadic PCs may have the HPT-JT syndrome or a variant of this syndrome. Thus, the strong association between *HRPT2* mutation and PC suggests that this molecular event has a pathogenic role for most sporadic PCs. It is worth noting that all the three studies included cases of unequivocal malignant tumors [41-43]. Most recent studies which included tumors classified as malignant on the basis of pathological criteria alone, without the requirement for clinical malignant behavior, reported a lower prevalence of *HRPT2* mutations [52]. Another mechanism of *HRPT2* gene inactivation, methylation of the promoter, has been reported in 2 of 11 PC [53]. *HRPT2* mutations are found, but only rarely, in sporadic benign parathyroid adenomas [24, 41, 43 54] suggesting that *HRPT2* mutations have a very limited, if any, role in the pathogenesis of typical sporadic adenomas. *HRPT2* encodes a 531 amino acids protein called parafibromin (parathyroid disease and fibro-osseous lesions), similar in homology (54%) to yeast protein Cdc73 (Cell Division Cycle protein 73) [24]. Like Cdc73, parafibromin is a component of RNA polymerase II/Paf1 complex, which is involved in the transcription elongation and RNA processing pathways [55-57]. Parafibromin is mostly a nuclear protein, that is evolutionary conserved [58-60], but it may also localize to the nucleolus [61].

The role of parafibromin as a tumor suppressor protein comes from the observation that parathyroid tumors carrying *HRPT2* mutations are frequently associated with loss of parafibromin expression or function. Over expression of wild type parafibromin in HEK-293 and NIH3T3 cells, but not its L64P mutant, which is implicated in PC, inhibited cell proliferation, by blocking cyclin D1 expression [62]. Thus, bi-allelic *HRPT2* inactivation is associated with loss of the inhibitory effect on cyclin D1 and neoplastic transformation in susceptible tissues [62]. In addition parafibromin has been shown to be involved in inducing apoptosis and inhibiting G1 to S transition of the cell cycle [59, 63]. The existence of a connection between parafibromin function and components of the transcription machinery is further supported by the fact that the *Drosophila* ortholog of human parafibromin, hyrax, binds to β-catenin/armadillo and is required for the nuclear transduction of the Wnt/Wingless pathway [64]. These observations establish the central role of parafibromin in the control of the cell cycle, and subsequently in determining cell fate and promoting tumorigenesis. The relationship of parafibromin with the complex network of nuclear components merits further investigation.

Table 7.1. Gene and related protein alterations in parathyroid carcinoma

Gene	Protein	Genetic abnormalities		Protein expression
		Mutation	LOH	
RB1	rb	absent	present	Decreased/absent
PRDA1	cyclin D1	ND[1]	ND	Increased
MKi67	Ki-67	?	?	Increased
BRAC2	BRAC2	ND	?	ND
CDKN1B	p27	ND	ND	Decreased
TP53	p53	?	?	Increased
CDC73/HRPT2	parafibromin	present	present	Decreased/absent
LGALS3	galectine-3	ND	ND	Increased
APC	APC	ND	ND	Decreased
CTNNB1	®-catenin	absent	ND	Normal
UCHL1	PGP9.5	ND	ND	Increased

[1] ND= not done. LOH= loss of heterozygosity.

Pathology

PC is mostly irregular, grayish-white and hard tumors, adherent to the surrounding tissues. Their size is usually over 3-cm in diameter and weight between 2 and 10 grams [4, 5, 65]. The finding of gross infiltration of contiguous structures strongly suggest the diagnosis of carcinoma. In 1973 Shanz and Castleman established a set of features of PC, including uniform sheets of cells (usually chief) arranged in a lobular pattern and separated by fibrous bands, mitotic figures, capsular or vascular invasion [66] (Figure 7.1). Capsular invasion is characterized by a “tongue-like” protrusion through the collagenous fibers and should be distinguished from pseudo invasion, due to “trapping” of tumor cells within the capsule, which can be found in adenoma [4, 67]. The criteria of vascular invasion have been differently defined according to whether capsular vessels or vessels in the surrounding tissues are involved [4, 67, 68]. Partial attachment of tumor cells to the wall of the vascular channel or thrombosis should also be present [4, 68]. The diagnostic value of capsular and vascular invasion is still debated. Some authors regard vascular invasion as virtually diagnostic of malignancy [4, 69]. Thus, controversy and diagnostic uncertainties still exist [4, 67, 68].

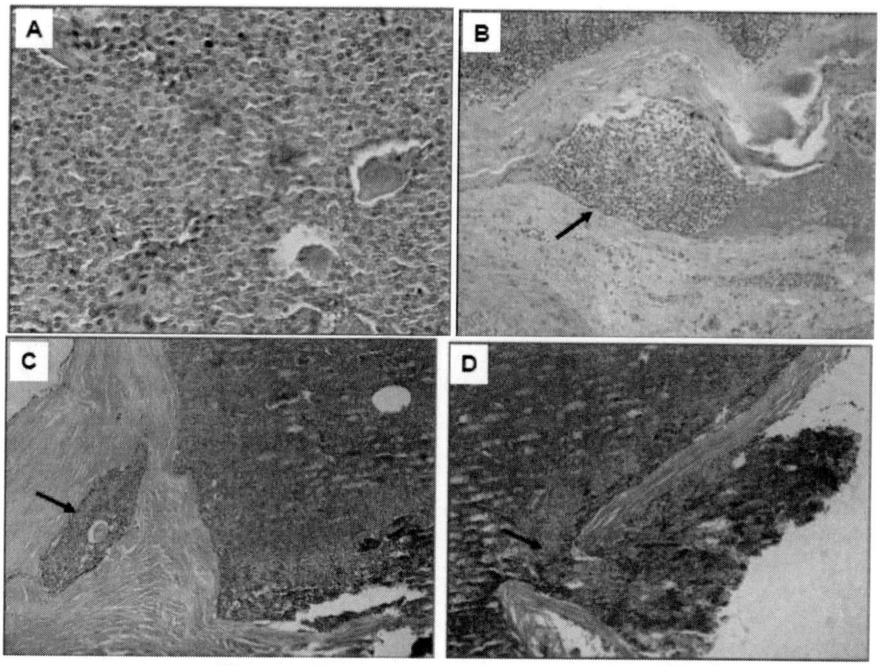

Figure 7.1. Pathologic features of parathyroid carcinoma. A) trabecular growth; B) vascular invasion (the arrow indicates the partial attachment of tumor cells to the wall of the vascular channel); C) pseudocapsular invasion (the arrow indicates the trapping of tumor cells within the capsule); D) capsular invasion (the arrow indicates a "tongue-like" protrusion through the collagenous fibers).

Some of the features pathognomonic of PC can also be found in a subset of parathyroid adenomas, which are referred as "atypical adenomas" [4]. Thus, as mentioned before, the distinction between benign and malignant parathyroid tumors cannot be definitively established at histology, unless there is evidence of invasion of extratumoral vessels, perineural spaces or surrounding tissues (Table 7.2). A full discussion of the pathology of PC is beyond the scope of this review. Immunohistochemistry is used to improve the accuracy of the diagnosis of PC (Table 7.1). An increased labeling of cell cycle-associated proliferation markers (Ki-67, cyclin D1) has been shown in PC compared to adenoma, but the overlap among benign and malignant tumors has limited its clinical utility [70-72]. A decreased expression of p27, an inhibitor of cyclin-dependent kinase, and abnormal Galectine-3 expression have been demonstrated in carcinomas [73, 74]. The association of low p27 and high Ki-67 labeling increases the likelihood of malignancy [73, 74]. Loss/altered expression of the calcium-sensing receptor (CaSR) is present in a subset of parathyroid adenoma and carcinoma and labeling of the CaSR has no diagnostic value [75, 76].

Following the demonstration that the *HRPT2* gene is involved in the pathogenesis of sporadic PC several studies have been performed to evaluate whether parafibromin immunostaining might have some diagnostic utility. A loss (total or focal) of staining has been reported in the large majority of clinically unequivocal PC and very rarely in adenomas [51, 76-81]. Cases of positive parafibromin staining in the presence of *HRPT2* mutation have also been reported in PC [79]. Limited data are available in equivocal cases, where this test would have a major diagnostic value. In this regard, it has been reported that negative parafibromin staining combined with *HRPT2* mutations is strongly associated with PC [51].

Table 7.2. Histological features of atypical adenoma and carcinoma

Parameter	Adenoma	Atypical adenoma	Carcinoma
Nuclear atypia	+	+	+
Mitosis	+/-	+	++
Macronuleoli	-	+	++
Necrosis	+	+	++
Fibrous band	+/-	++	++
Trabecular growth	-	++	++
Pseudocapsular invasion	-	+	+
Vascular invasion [1]	-	-	+
Capsular invasion	-	-	+
Tissue invasion	-	-	+

[1]The criteria of vascular invasion have been differently defined according to whether capsular vessels or vessels in the surrounding tissues are involved [4, 67, 68]. Partial attachment of tumor cells to the wall of the vascular channel or thrombosis should also be present.

More recently Juhlin et al. have evaluated two additional molecular markers in PC. The staining of the protein gene product 9.5 (PGP9.5), which is increased in PC, has shown promise, with a greater sensitivity for detecting malignancy compared to that of parafibromin [82]. Loss of staining of tumor suppressor adenomatous polyposis coli (APC) has been found in the majority of PC but not in adenoma [83]. Interestingly, APC staining was retained in parathyroid adenoma with *HRPT2* mutations and loss of parafibromin expression, suggesting a greater specificity.

It is important to emphasize that the diagnostic potential of these tests hinges on their common presence in PC and their rarity in benign disease. Since benign parathyroid disease is so much more common than PC, a test that has a detectable detection rate in benign parathyroid disease (even if low) would have limited clinical utility. The positive predictive value of the test may be increased, therefore, if the *HRPT2* gene/parafibromin analysis is restricted to cases that are equivocal. The combined findings of negative parafibromin staining and *HRPT2* gene abnormalities increase the likelihood of a malignancy (51, 81). Based on this reasoning, it seems appropriate to evaluate all parathyroid tumors in which the diagnosis is uncertain for abnormalities of both the *HRPT2* gene and its product, parafibromin.

Clinical Presentation

The clinical manifestations of PC are mostly due to the effects of markedly elevated serum PTH and calcium, rather than to local infiltration or metastases [2-4]. Occasionally PCs may be nonfunctional [84].

The typical clinical picture is characterized by renal involvement (nephrocalcinosis, nephrolithiasis, impaired renal function) in up to 80% of patients and bone involvement (osteitis fibrosa cystica, subperiostal resorption, "salt and pepper" skull, diffuse osteopenia) in up to 90% [2-4]. On physical examination most patients with PC have a palpable neck mass. Renal colic is a frequent presenting complaint. Other symptoms include fatigue, muscle weakness, nausea, polydipsia and polyuria, depression, bone pain, and fractures. Recurrent severe pancreatitis, peptic ulcer disease, and anemia can also occur. None of these features is pathognomonic of malignancy. In the majority of cases, the diagnosis of PC is made only in retrospect when hypercalcemia recurs due to local spread of tumor or distant metastases. PC can be misdiagnosed as thyroid or thymic carcinoma because of locally advanced disease (palpable neck mass, dysphagia, hoarseness due to laryngeal nerve palsy). Immunohistochemistry for PTH, thyroglobulin, thyroid transcription factor 1 and calcitonin may help ascertain the correct diagnosis.

Despite these clinical features which may suggest a malignant tumor, the challenge to the clinicians rests upon differentiating between PHPT due to PC and that due to its much more common benign counterpart. The occurrence of metastases is the only unequivocal criterion of malignancy that is generally accepted, but they usually occur late in the course of the disease. Additional features could suggest a malignant rather than a benign etiology (Table 7.3):

A summary of the typical features differentiating PC from adenoma is reported in Table 7.1.

Recent data demonstrate that in some patients with PC a new PTH moiety is overproduced, i.e., a N-terminal PTH molecule (N-PTH), distinct from the intact human 1-84 PTH, which is recognized in a 3rd-generation assay of "whole" PTH [85]. The clinical implications of this finding in PC await additional studies in a large series of patients with an emphasis on N-PTH's biological activity. Serum alkaline phosphatase is also higher in patients with PC than in those with adenoma, in whom serum levels are generally close to the upper limit of the normal range. 〈 and ®-subunits of hCG may be elevated in patients with PC but not in those with benign tumors [86]. PC should also be suspected in a hypercalcemic patient without a history of prior neck surgery, who presents with recurrent laryngeal nerve palsy.

Table 7.3. Clinical characteristics used in the differential diagnosis between parathyroid adenoma and carcinoma

	Adenoma	Carcinoma
Female:male ratio	3-4:1	01:01
Average age at diagnosis (yr)	55	48
Serum calcium (mg/dl)	<13	>14
Serum PTH	Elevated	Markedly Elevated
Symptoms of hypercalcemia	Present	Present
Palpable cervical lesion	Rare	Common
Concomitant bone and renal involvement	Rare	Common

a) *male gender*. There is no sex preference, whereas the male:female ratio in benign PHPT is 3-4:1.
b) *relatively young age*. The average age of PC a patient at diagnosis is in the mid-40s, about 10 yr younger than the usual patient with adenoma.
c) *markedly elevated serum calcium and PTH*. Most patients with parathyroid adenomas have serum calcium levels 13 mg/dl whereas the calcium levels in patients with PC are usually in excess of 14-15 mg/dl. As might be expected, PTH levels are markedly elevated in patients with PC; on the other hand in those with adenomas PTH levels may be only slightly elevated.
d) *bone and renal involvement*: The combination of both renal and bone manifestations at the time of presentation suggests the possibility of PC. In benign PHPT, clinically overt bone disease is no longer commonly seen, and concomitant skeletal and renal involvement is uncommon.
e) *size of the parathyroid lesion at initial surgery*. Carcinoma size is usually over 3-cm in diameter.

PC shares many clinical features with acute PHPT, sometimes called "parathyroid crisis" (marked elevations of serum calcium and PTH). Although the distinction between the two entities is not possible preoperatively, it is important to bear in mind the diagnosis of malignancy because the surgical approach differs.

When benign PHPT presents with markedly elevated serum calcium concentrations and overt target organ involvement, a clinical phenotype that was historically common but is now infrequently seen in most countries, the clinical distinction between benign and malignant disease may be difficult. However, it is preferable to have a high index of suspicion for PC when these features are present than to miss the opportunity for surgical cure (more extended surgery) by failing to consider it in the differential diagnosis.

Natural History

PC has a rather low malignant potential and typically runs an indolent, albeit progressive course [2-4]. At initial presentation, involvement of regional lymph nodes (5 %) or distant sites (2%) is rarely found [87].

PC generally recurs locally and spreads to contiguous neck structures. Metastases occur late in the course of the disease, involving cervical nodes (30%) and lung (40%), and, less frequently, liver (10%). Occasionally metastases in bone, pleura, pericardium and pancreas have been reported.

The identification of germline *HRPT2* mutations in about one third of patients with apparently sporadic PC [28, 42, 43, 51] suggests that a subset of these patients might have the HPT-JT syndrome or variant thereof. This finding is relevant for the follow up. When a recurrence of hypercalcemia occurs in such patients, in addition to the likelihood that the original PC has recurred, a new parathyroid tumour should be carefully sought, because multiglandular involvement can develop in patients with HPT-JT syndrome. Surveillance for renal and jaw lesions is also indicated. Moreover, the relatives of a patient with PC carrying a germline *HRPT2* mutation are susceptible to the development of PC or other manifestation of HPT-JT syndrome [49, 50]. Therefore, monitoring of family members is recommended.

Management and Prognosis

Surgery

Surgery is the only effective treatment of PC and consists of complete resection of the primary lesion at the time of initial operation [2, 7]. The most effective therapy is *en bloc* resection [88-91]. The standard *en bloc* resection consists of the removal of the parathyroid tumor along with the ipsilateral thyroid lobe. Holmes et al. suggested a more aggressive approach including ipsilateral thyroidectomy and isthmusectomy, skeletonization of the trachea, excision of the neighboring muscles and removal of the recurrent laryngeal nerve, if involved [92]. Care should be taken during dissection to avoid rupture of the capsule, as cell spillage is associated with multifocal recurrences and persistent hypercalcemia. Tracheoesphageal, paratracheal, and upper mediastinal lymph nodes should be excised, but an extensive lateral neck dissection is indicated only when there is spread to the anterior cervical nodes. There are only a few anecdotal reports of parathyroid cancer spread to lymph nodes [93] Thus, preoperative suspicion and intraoperative recognition of a potential malignant lesion are of great importance for designing the surgical strategy. Patient with a clinical presentation suggestive of PC warrant thorough exploration of all four parathyroid glands, as PC has been report to coexist with benign adenomas or hyperplasia [16, 26].

When the diagnosis is made in the early postoperative period on the basis of pathology, as most usually happens, re-exploration of the neck is indicated, particularly if the pathology showed extensive vascular or capsular invasion or if hypercalcemia persists. When the above histological features are absent, the patient is normocalcaemic and the diagnosis of PC is only based on the pathology, the simple complete resection of the tumors may be curative. Such a patient should be monitored closely with serum calcium and PTH levels measurements.

Following parathyroidectomy patients may experience the "hungry bone syndrome", characterized by symptomatic hypocalcemia due to the deposition of calcium and phosphorus in the bones. Hypocalcemia may be severe and require administration of intravenous calcium. Oral calcium and calcitriol should be simultaneously started and maintained for several weeks when 'hungary bone syndrome' is present. Afterwards the administration of calcium and calcitriol can be stopped, because of the recovery of the remaining parathyroid glands. Thereafter, serum calcium and PTH should be monitored every three months.

Despite curative resection, recurrence of PC occurs in up to 50% of cases, most commonly 2-3 years after the initial surgery, but a prolonged disease-free interval of 20 years has been reported [2-4, 93]. Imaging studies should be performed in all patients before re-operation. Neck ultrasonography is fast and can detect cervical recurrences. Technetium 99m-sestamibi can visualize local recurrences and distant metastases [95]. It can be also used for the intraoperative localization of abnormal parathyroid tissues [96]. Computerized tomography and magnetic resonance imaging are useful adjuncts to ultrasonography in the evaluation of the neck and are superior for detection of metastases in the chest or abdomen. Fine-needle aspiration of a suspicious lesion with measurement of PTH in the aspirate should be used with caution, if at all, to avoid seeding the needle track with deposits of malignant cells [97, 98]. Arteriography and selective venous sampling for PTH measurement can be used in selected cases when non-invasive studies are negative. The management of recurrent or metastatic PC is primarily surgical [2-4, 7, 87-89, 94, 99]. Recurrences in the neck should be treated with wide resections, including the regional lymph nodes and other involved structures. Accessible distant metastases, particularly in the presence of localized metastatic disease, should also be excised, if possible. Even a small tumor may produce a sufficient amount of PTH to cause hypercalcemia, and although resection is rarely curative, its removal may result in periods of normocalcemia ranging from months to years [7, 81].

Chemotherapy

The rarity of PC precludes any prospective study to examine the effects of chemotherapy and most knowledge on this matter derives from case reports. Several regimens have been attempted, using nitrogen mustard, vincristine, cyclophosphamide, and actinomycin D, and adriamycin alone or in combination with cyclophosphamide and 5-fluorouracil, but none of them proved to be effective [100, 101]. Currently, there is no role for chemotherapy in the management of patients with PC.

Radiotherapy

Radiation therapy has not had significant effect shown in a large series in the management of invasive PC. An apparent cure has been reported in a patient with tracheal invasion. Recent case series have suggested the use of irradiation as adjuvant therapy and a disease-free survival at a median follow-up period of 60 months in four patients who received postoperative radiotherapy [91,102, 103]. A lower local recurrence rate has been reported if adjuvant radiation was given after surgery, independent of the type of operation and the disease stage [104, 105]

Management of Hypercalcemia

When PC has became widely metastatic and surgical options are exhausted, clinical management turns to controlling hypercalcemia. Saline infusion and loop diuretics are often used, but, in the majority of cases potent intravenous bisphosphonates (pamidronate and zoledronate) are used. They may transiently control hypercalcemia, but patients frequently become refractory to them. Plycamicin is effective, but the response is transient, and repeated courses may be associated with toxicity. Gallium nitrate is also an effective hypocalcaemic drug, but its use is limited by nephrotoxicity. Calcitonin may reduce transiently serum calcium in patients with PC. Octreotide, the long-acting somatostatin analogue, has also been reported to inhibit PTH secretion in a woman with PC metastatic to bone [106]. Because the primary cause of death is PTH-driven hypercalcemia, rather than direct tumor invasion and spread, one approach is to target the parathyroid cell CASR. Calcimimetics, allosteric modulators of the CASR, directly reduce parathyroid cell hormone secretion by binding to the CASR on parathyroid cells, increasing their sensitivity to extracellular calcium [107]. A first generation calcimimetic, R-568, was used for 2 years in a patient with metastatic PC with controlled hypercalcemia [108]. R-568 has been replaced by cinacalcet, a more potent second-generation agent with a longer half-life. Cinacalcet effectively reduced hypercalcemia in about two-thirds of patients with inoperable PC [109, 110] (Figure 7.2). Nausea and vomiting were the most common adverse events, and required discontinuation of drug in some cases.

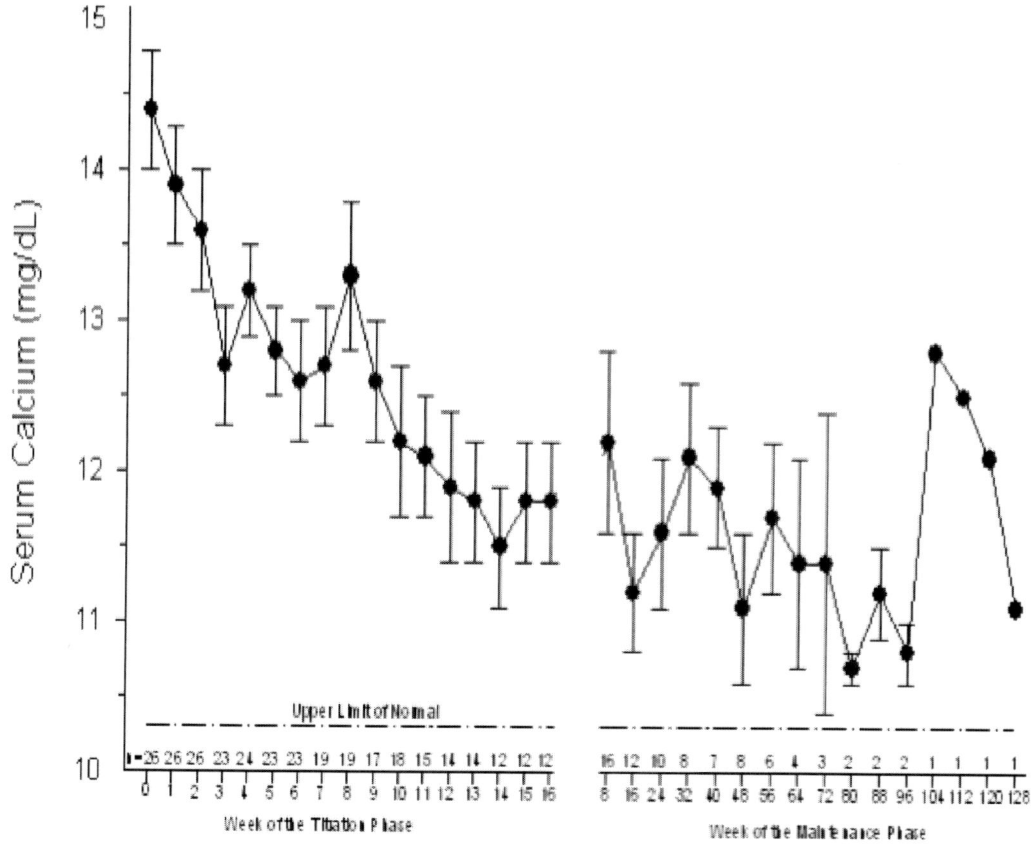

Figure 7.2. Reduction in serum calcium concentration in parathyroid cancer with cinacalcet. Subjects were given cinacalcet in increasing doses, up to 90 mg four times daily during the titration phase. The average serum calcium fell from 14.5±0.4 mg/dL to 12.4±0.4 mg/dL (P=0.001). (Reprinted from Marcocci C, Cetani F, Rubin MR, Silverberg SJ, Pinchera A, Bilezikian JP 2008 Parathyroid carcinoma. J Bone Miner Res 23:1869-80; Copyright 2008, *Journal of Bone and Mineral Research*).

There are no data suggesting that cinacalcet alters the course of the PC itself. Cinacalcet therefore represents an important new option for management of intractable hypercalcemia in patients with inoperable disease. Furthermore, unlike other options for treatment of hypercalcemia, this agent can be used in patients with the renal impairment so common in patients with longstanding PC. Another novel and promising approach is anti-PTH immunotherapy. A positive response has been observed in a patient with metastatic PC immunized with a mixture of human and bovine PTH peptides [111, 112]. Recently, a monoclonal antibody to PTH has been used for the treatment of PC [113]. Dendritic cell-immunotherapy may also be applicable to induce a T-cell immune response [114].

Prognosis

The prognosis of PC is quite variable and depends from its early recognition and complete excision of the tumor at initial surgery. The mean time to recurrence is usually 3 yr, although intervals of up to 20 yr have been reported [2, 4, 92]. When recurrence occurs, complete cure is unlikely, although prolonged survival is still common with palliative surgery. Five-year survival rates vary from 40% to 86% and the National Surveillance, Epidemiology and End Results database recently reported a 10-yr survival rate of 67.8% [114].

Conclusion

The diagnosis of PC is often not clear at the time of presentation, even though some clinical features may be helpful. The distinction between benign and malignant parathyroid tumours cannot be definitively established at histology, unless there is evidence of invasion of extratumoral vessels, perineural spaces or surrounding tissues. Recently, genetic and immunohistological analyses have shown promise at helping with histological diagnosis. The disease is indolent but progressive. The best opportunity to cure PC is to diagnose it before or at the time of parathyroid surgery and for the tumor to be completely removed at the time of the initial operation. Removal of local recurrences and distant metastases can provide short and long term control. Chemotherapy has not been shown to be of benefit and radiotherapy has anecdotal reports of effectiveness at managing recurrent and persistent disease. Intravenous bisphosphomates and cinacalcet can be used to target the consequence of the disease (hypercalcemia) rather than the disease itself when surgical options are exhausted.

References

[1] Silverberg SJ, Bilezikian JP Primary Hyperparathyroidism 2008 In:Rosen JF (Ed) *Primer on the Metabolic Bone Diseases and Disorders of Mineral Metabolism*, 7th Edition , p. 302-306.

[2] Marcocci C, Cetani F, Rubin MR, Silverberg SJ, Pinchera A, Bilezikian JP 2008 Parathyroid carcinoma. *J. Bone Miner. Res.* 23:1869-80.

[3] Shane E 2001 Clinical Review 122: parathyroid carcinoma. *J. Clin. Endocrinol. Metab.* 2:485-493.

[4] De Lellis RA 2005 Parathyroid carcinoma. An overview. *Adv. Anat. Pathol.* 12:53-61.

[5] Bondenson L, Grimelius L, DeLellis RA, Lloyd R, Akerstrom G, Larsson C, Arnold A, Eng C, Shane E, Bilezikian JP 2004. *Parathyroid carcinoma*. In: DeLellis RA, Lloyd RV, Heitz PU, Eng (eds.) C Pathology and genetics. Tumors of endocrine organs. WHO Classification of Tumours, IARC Press, Lyon, France, pp 124-27.

[6] Cetani F, Pardi E, Banti C, Borsari S, Ambrogini E, Vignali E, Cianferotti L, Viccica G, Pinchera A, Marcocci C 2008 *HRPT2* gene analysis and diagnosis of parathyroid carcinoma, *Expert Rev. Endocrinol. Metab.* 3:377-389.

[7] Shane E 2001 Parathyroid carcinoma. In: Bilezikian JP, Marcus R, Levine MA (eds.) The Parathyroids. Basic and Clinical Concepts, 2nd ed., Academic Press, San Diego, CA, USA, pp 515-25.

[8] Hundahl SA, Fleming ID, Fremgen AM, Menck HR 1999 Two hundred eighty-six cases of parathyroid carcinoma treated in the U.S. between 1985-1999: A National Cancer Database report. The American College of Surgeons Commission on Cancer and the American Cancer Society. *Cancer,* 86:538-44.

[9] Favia G, Lumachi F, Polistina F, D'Amico DF 1998 Parathyroid carcinoma: sixteen new cases and suggestions for correct management. *World J. Surg.* 22:1225-1230.

[10] Obara T, Fujimoto Y 1991 Diagnosis and treatment of patients with parathyroid carcinoma: An update and review. *Word J. Surg.* 15:738-744.

[11] Ireland J, Fleming S, Levison D, Cattell W, Baker L 1985 Parathyroid carcinoma associated with chronic renal failure and previous radiotherapy to the neck. *J. Clin. Pathol.* 38:1114-1118.

[12] Christmas TJ, Chapple CR, Noble JG, Milroy EJ, Cowie AG 1988 Hyperparathyroidism after neck irradiation. *Br. J. Surg.* 75:873-874.

[13] Cohen J, Gierlowski TC, Schneider AB 1990 A prospective study of hyperparathyroidism in individuals exposed to radiation in childhood. *JAMA* 264:581-584.

[14] Schneider AB, Gierlowski TC, Shore-Freedman E, Stovall M, Ron E, Lubin J 1995 Dose-response relationships for radiation-induced hyperparathyroidism. *J. Clin. Endocrinol. Metab.* 80:254-257.

[15] Rasmuson T, Damber L, Johansson L, Johansson R, Larsson LG 2002 Increased incidence of parathyroid adenomas following X-ray treatment of benign diseases in the cervical spine in adult patients. *Clin. Endocrinol.* (Oxf) 57:731-734.

[16] Berland Y, Olmer M, Lebreuil G, Grisoli J 1982 Parathyroid carcinoma, adenoma and hyperplasia in a case of chronic renal insufficiency on dialysis. *Clin. Nephrol.* 18:154-158.

[17] Boyle NH, Ogg CS, Hartley RB, Owen WJ 1999 Parathyroid carcimoma secondary to prolonged hyperplasia in chronic renal failure and celiac disease. *Eur. J. Surg. Oncol.* 25:100-103.

[18] Streeten EA, Weinstein LS, Norton JA, Mulvihill JJ, White BJ, Friedman E, JaffeG, Brandi ML, Stewart K, Zimering MB, Spiegel AM, Aurbach GD, Marx SJ 1992 Studies in a kindred with parathyroid carcinoma. *J. Clin. Endocrinol. Metab.* 75:362-366.

[19] Wassif WS, Moniz CF, Friedman E, Wong S, Weber G, Nordenskjöld M, Peters TJ, Larsson C 1993 Familial isolated hyperparathyroidism: a distinct genetic entity with an increased risk of parathyroid cancer. *J. Clin. Endocrinol. Metab.* 77:1485-1489.

[20] Yoshimoto K, Endo H, Tsuyuguchi M, Tanaka C, Kimura T, Iwahana H, Kato G, Sano T, Itakura 1998 Familial isolated primary hyperparathyroidism with parathyroid carcinomas: clinical and molecular features. *Clin. Endocrinol.* (Oxf) 48:67-72.

[21] Marx SJ, Simonds WF, Agarwal SK, Burns AL, Weinstein LS, Cochran C, Skarulis, MC, Spiegel AM, Libutti SK, Alexander HR Jr, Chen CC, Chang R, Chandrasekharappa, SC, Collins FS 2002 Hyperparathyroidism in hereditary syndromes: special expressions and special managements. *J. Bone Miner. Res.* 17 (Suppl 2):N37-43.

[22] Chen JD, Morrison C, Zhang C, Kahnoski K, Carpten JD, Teh BT 2003 Hyperparathyroidism-jaw tumour syndrome. *J. Intern Med.* 253:634-642.

[23] Mallette LE, Malini S, Rappaport MP, Kirkland JL 1987 Familial cystic parathyroid adenomatosis. *Ann. Intern Med.* 107:54-60.

[24] Carpten JD, Robbins CM, Villablanca A, Forsberg L, Presciuttini S, Bailey-Wilson J, Simonds WF, Gillanders EM, Kennedy AM, Chen JD, Agarwal SK, Sood R, Jones MP, Moses TY, Haven C, Petillo D, Leotlela PD, Harding B, Cameron D, Pannett AA, Hoog A, Heath,H. 3rd, James-Newton LA, Robinson B, Zarbo RJ, Cavaco BM, Wassif W, Perrier ND, Rosen IB, Kristoffersson U, Turnpenny PD, Farnebo LO, Besser GM, Jackson CE, Morreau H, Trent JM, Thakker RV, Marx SJ, The BT, Larsson C, Hobbs MR 2002 HRPT2, encoding parafibromin, is mutated in hyperparathyroidism-jaw tumors syndrome. *Nature Genetics* 32:676-680.

[25] Simonds WF, James-Newton LA, Agarwal SK, Yang B, Skarulis MC, Hendy GN, Marx SJ 2002 Familial isolated hyperparathyroidism: clinical and genetic characteristics of 36 kindreds. *Medicine* (Baltimore) 81:1-26.

[26] Dionisi S, Minisola S, Pepe J, De Geronimo S, Paglia F, Memeo L, Fitzpatrick LA 2002 Concurrent parathyroid adenomas and carcinoma in the setting of multiple endocrine neoplasia type 1: presentation as hypercalcemic crisis. *Mayo Clin. Proc.* 77:866-869.

[27] Agha A, Carpenter R, Bhattacharya S, Edmonson SJ, Carlsen E, Monson JP 2007 Parathyroid carcinoma in multiple endocrine neoplasia type 1 (MEN1) syndrome: Two case reports of an unrecognized entity. *J. Endocrinol. Invest.* 30:145-149.

[28] Haven CJ, van Puijenbroek M, Tan MH, Teh BT, Fleuren GJ, van Wezel T, Morreau H 2007 Identification of MEN1 and HRPT2 somatic mutations in paraffin-embedded (sporadic) parathyroid carcinomas. *Clin. Endocrinol.* (Oxf) 67:370-376.

[29] Shih RY, Fackler S, Maturo S, True MW, Brennan J, Wells D. 2009 Parathyroid carcinoma in multiple endocrine neoplasia type 1 with a classic germline mutation. Endocr. Pract. 15:567-572.

[30] Jenkins PJ, Satta MA, Simmgen M, Drake WM, Williamson C, Lowe DG, Britton K, Chew SL, Thakker RV, Besser GM 1997 Metastatic parathyroid carcinoma in the MEN2A syndrome. *Clin. Endocrinol.* (Oxf). 47:747-751.

[31] Arnold A, Shattuck TM, Mallya SM, Krebs LJ, Costa J, Gallagher J, Wild Y, Saucier K. Molecular pathogenesis of primary hyperparathyroidism 2002 *J. Bone Miner. Res.* 17 Suppl 2:N30-36.

[32] Cetani F, Pardi E, Borsari S, Lemmi M, Ambrogini E, Vignali E, Cianferotti L, Pinchera M 2006 Parathyroid tumorigenesis. *Clin. Cases Min. Bone Metab.* 3:123-131.

[33] Cryns VL, Thor A, Xu HJ, Hu SX, Wierman ME, Vickery AL Jr, Benedict WF, Arnold A 1994 Loss of the retinoblastoma tumor-suppressor gene in parathyroid carcinoma. *N. Engl. J. Med.* 330:757-761.

[34] Dotzenrath C, The T, Farnebo F, Cupisti K, Svensson A, Toell A, Goretzki P, Larsson C 1996 Allelic loss of the retinoblastoma tumor suppressor gene: a marker for aggressive parathyroid tumors? *J. Clin. Endocrinol. Metab.* 8:3194-3196.

[35] Pearce SH, Trump D, Wooding W, Sheppard MN, Clayton RN, Thakker RV 1996 Loss of heterozygosity study at the retinoblastoma and breast cancer susceptibility (BRCA2) loci in pituitary, parathyroid, pancreatic and carcinoid tumors. *Clin. Endocrinol.* (Oxf) 45:195-200.

[36] Cetani F, Pardi E, Viacava P, Pollina GD, Fanelli G, Picone A, Borsari S, Gazzerro E, Miccoli P, Berti P, Pinchera A, Marcocci C 2004 A reappraisal of the Rb1 gene abnormalities in the diagnosis of parathyroid cancer. *Clinical Endocrinology*, 60 99-106.

[37] Shattuck TM, Kim TS, Costa J, Yandell DW, Imanishi Y, Palanisamy N, Gaz RD, Shoback D, Clark OH, Monchik JM, Wierman ME, Hollenberg A, Tojo K, Chaganti, RS, Arnold A 2003 Mutational analyses of RB and BRCA2 as candidate tumour suppressor genes in parathyroid carcinoma. *Clin. Endocrinol.* (Oxf) 59:180-89.

[38] Cryns, VL, Rubio, MP, Thor, AD, Louis, DN, Arnold, A 1994 p53 abnormalities in human parathyroid carcinoma. *Journal of Clinical Endocrinology and Metabolism* 78:1320-1324.

[39] Vargas MP, Vargas HI, Kleiner DE, Merino MJ. The role of prognostic markers (MiB-1, RB, and bcl-2) in the diagnosis of parathyroid tumors. *Mod. Pathol.* 1997,10:12-7.

[40] Cetani F, Pardi E, Banti C, Collecchi P, Viacava P, Borsari S, Fanelli G, Naccarato AG, Saponaro F, Berti P, Miccoli P, Pinchera A, Marcocci C. 2010 Beta-catenin activation is not involved in sporadic parathyroid carcinomas and adenomas. *Endocr. Relat. Cancer* 17:1-6.

[41] Howell VM, Haven CJ, Kahnoski K, Khoo SK, Petillo D, Chen J, Fleuren GJ, Robinson BG, Delbridge LW, Philips J, Nelson AE, Krause U, Hammje K, Dralle H, Hoang-Vu C, Gimm O, Marsh DJ, Morreau H, Teh BT 2003 HRPT2 mutations are associated with malignancy in sporadic parathyroid tumours. *J. Med. Genet.* 40:657-663.

[42] Shattuck TM, Valimaki S, Obara T, Gaz RD, Clark OH, Shoback D, Wierman ME, Tojo K, Robbins CM, Carpten JD Farnebo LO, Larsson C, Arnold A 2003 Somatic and germ-line mutations of the HRPT2 gene in sporadic parathyroid carcinoma. *N. Engl. J. Med.* 349:1722-1729.

[43] Cetani F, Pardi E, Borsari S, Viacava P, Dipollina G, Cianferotti L, Ambrogini E, Gazzerro E, Colussi G, Berti P, Miccoli P, Pinchera A, Marcocci C 2004 Genetic analyses of the HRPT2 gene in primary hyperparathyroidism: germline and somatic mutations in familial and sporadic parathyroid tumors. *J. Clin. Endocrinol. Metab.* 89:5583-5591.

[44] Simonds WF, Robbins CM, Agarwal SK, Hendy GN, Carpten JD, Marx SJ 2004 Familial isolated hyperparathyroidism is rarely caused by germline mutation in HRPT2, the gene for the hyperparathyroidism-jaw tumor syndrome. *J. Clin. Endocrinol. Metab.* 89:96-102.

[45] Warner J, Epstein M, Sweet A, Singh D, Burgess J, Stranks S, Hill P, Perry-Keene D, Learoyd D, Robinson B, Birdsey P, Mackenzie E, Teh BT, Prins JB, Cardinal J 2004 Genetic testing in familial isolated hyperparathyroidism: unexpected results and their implications. *J. Med. Genet.* 41:155-160.

[46] Villablanca A, Calender A, Forsberg L, Höög A, Cheng JD, Petillo D, Bauters C, Kahnoski K, Ebeling T, Salmela P, Richardson AL, Delbridge L, Meyrier A, Proye C, Carpten JD, Teh BT, Robinson BG, Larsson C 2004. Germline and de novo mutations in the HRPT2 tumour suppressor gene in familial isolated hyperparathyroidism (FIHP). *J. Med. Genet.* 41:e32.

[47] Bradley KJ, Cavaco BM, Bowl MR, Harding B, Cranston T, Fratter C, Besser GM, Conceição Pereira M, Davie MW, Dudley N, Leite V, Sadler GP, Seller A, Thakker RV 2006 Parafibromin mutations in hereditary hyperparathyroidism syndromes and parathyroid tumours. *Clin. Endocrinol.* (Oxf) 64:299-306.

[48] Mizusawa N, Uchino S, Iwata T, Tsuyuguchi M, Suzuki Y, Mizukoshi T, Yamashita Y, Sakurai A, Suzuki S, Beniko M, Tahara H, Fujisawa M, Kamata N, Fujisawa K, Yashiro T, Nagao D, Golam HM, Sano T, Noguchi S, Yoshimoto K 2006 Genetic analyses in patients with familial isolated hyperparathyroidism and hyperparathyroidism-jaw tumour syndrome. *Clin. Endocrinol.* (Oxf) 65:9-16.

[49] Guarnieri V, Scillitani A, Muscarella LA, Battista C, Bonfitto N, Bisceglia M, Minisola S, Mascia ML, D'Agruma L, Cole DE 2006 Diagnosis of parathyroid tumors in familial isolated hyperparathyroidism with HRPT2 mutation: implications for cancer surveillance. *J. Clin. Endocrinol. Metab.* 91:2827-2832.

[50] Kelly TG, Shattuck TM, Reyes-Mugica M, Stewart AF, Simonds WF, Udelsman R, Arnold A, Carpenter TO 2006 Surveillance for early detection of aggressive parathyroid disease: carcinoma and atypical adenoma in familial isolated hyperparathyroidism associated with a germline HRPT2 mutation. *J. Bone Miner. Res.* 21:1666-1671.

[51] Cetani F, Ambrogini E, Viacava P, Pardi E, Fanelli G, Naccarato AG, Borsari S, Lemmi M, Berti P, Miccoli P, Pinchera A, Marcocci C 2007 Should parafibromin staining replace HRPT2 gene analysis as an additional tool for histologic diagnosis of parathyroid carcinoma? *Eur. J. Endocrinol.* 156:547-554.

[52] Haven CJ, van Puijenbroek M, Tan MH, Teh BT, Fleuren GJ, van Wezel T, Morreau H 2007 Identification of MEN1 and HRPT2 somatic mutations in paraffin-embedded (sporadic) parathyroid carcinomas. *Clin. Endocrinol.* (Oxf) 67:370-376.

[53] Hewitt KM, Sharma PK, Samowitz W, Hobbs M 2007 Aberrant methylation of the HRPT2 gene in parathyroid carcinoma. *Ann. Otol. Rhinol. Laryngol.* 116:928-933.

[54] Krebs LJ, Shattuck TM and Arnold A 2005 HRPT2 mutational analysis of typical sporadic parathyroid adenomas. *J. Clin. Endocrinol. Metab.* 90:5015-5017.

[55] Chaudhary K, Deb S, Moniaux N, Ponnusamy MP, Batra SK 2007 Human RNA polymerase II-associated factor complex: dysregulation in cancer. *Oncogene* 26:7499-7507.

[56] Rozenblatt-Rosen O, Hughes CM, Nannepaga SJ, Shanmugam KS, Copeland TD, Guszczynski T, Resau JH, Meyerson M 2005 The parafibromin tumor suppressor protein is part of a human Paf1 complex. *Mol. Cell Biol*. 25 612-620.

[57] Yart A, Gstaiger M, Wirbelauer C, Pecnik M, Anastasiou D, Hess D, Krek W 2005 The HRPT2 tumor suppressor gene product parafibromin associates with human PAF1 and RNA polymerase II. *Mol. Cell Biol.* 25 5052-5060.

[58] Hahn MA, Marsh DJ 2005 Identification of a functional bipartite nuclear localization signal in the tumor suppressor parafibromin. *Oncogene* 24 6241-6248.

[59] Lin L, Czapiga M, Nini L, Zhang JH, Simonds WF 2007 Nuclear localization of the parafibromin tumor suppressor protein implicated in the hyperparathyroidism-jaw tumor syndrome enhances its proapoptotic function. *Mol. Cancer. Res* 5:183-193.

[60] Bradley KJ, Bowl MR, Williams SE, Ahmad BN, Partridge CJ, Patmanidi AL,Kennedy AM, Loh NY, Thakker RV 2007 Parafibromin is a nuclear protein with a functional monopartite nuclear localization signal. *Oncogene,* 26:1213-1221.

[61] Hahn MA, Marsh DJ 2007 Nucleolar localization of parafibromin is mediated by three nucleolar localization signals. *FEBS. Lett*. 581: 5070-5074.

[62] Woodard GE, Lin L, Zhang JH, Agarwal SK, Marx SJ, Simonds WF 2005 Parafibromin, product of the hyperparathyroidism-jaw tumor syndrome gene HRPT2, regulates cyclin D1/PRAD1 expression. *Oncogene* 24:1272-1276.

[63] Zhang C, Kong D, Tan MH, Pappas DL Jr, Wang PF, Chen J, Farber L, Zhang N, Koo, HM, Weinreich M, Williams BO, Teh BT 2006 Parafibromin inhibits cancer cell growth and causes G1 phase arrest. *Biochem. Biophys. Res. Commun*. 350:17-24.

[64] Mosimann C, Hausmann G, Basler K 2006 Parafibromin/Hyrax activates Wnt/Wg target gene transcription by direct association with beta-catenin/Armadillo. *Cell,* 125 327-341.

[65] Wang CA, Gaz RD 1985 Natural history of parathyroid carcinoma. Diagnosis, treatment and results. *Am. J. Surg*. 149:522-527.

[66] Schantz A, Castleman B 1973 Parathyroid carcinoma. A study of 70 cases. *Cancer* 31:600-605.

[67] LiVolsi VA 1985 Pathology of the parathyroid gland. In: Barnes L (ed.) Surgical Pathology of the Head and Neck, Marcel Dekker Inc.New York, pp 1487.

[68] Apel RL, Asa SL 2002 The Parathyroid Glands. In LiVolsi VA, Asa SL (eds.) Endocrine Pathology, Churchill Livingstone, Phipadelphia, pp 103-147.

[69] Smith JF, Coombs RRH 1984 Histological diagnosis of carcinoma of the parathyroid gland. *J. Clin. Pathol*. 37:1370-1378.

[70] Abbona GC, Papotti M, Gasparri G, Bussolati G 1995 Proliferative activity in parathyroid tumors as detected by Ki-67 immunostaining. *Hum. Pathol*. 26:135-138.

[71] Farnebo F, Auer G, Farnebo LO, Teh BT, Twigg S, Aspenblad U, Thompson NW, Grimelius L, Larsson C, Sandelin K 1999 Evaluation of retinoblastoma and Ki-67 immunostaining as diagnostic markers of benign and malignant parathyroid disease. *World J. Surg*. 23:68-74.

[72] Naccarato AG, Marcocci C, Miccoli P, Bonadio AG, Cianferotti L, Vignali E, Cipollini G, Viacava P 1998 Bcl-2, p53 and MIB-1 expression in normal and neoplastic parathyroid tissues. *J. Endocrinol. Invest* 21:136-141.

[73] Erickson LA, Jin L, Wollan P, Thompson GB, van Heerden JA, Lloyd RV 1999 Parathyroid hyperplasia, adenomas, and carcinomas: differential expression of p27Kip1 protein. *Am. J. Surg. Pathol*. 23:288-295.

[74] Bergero N, De Pompa R, Sacerdote C, Gasparri G, Volante M, Bussolati G, Papotti M 2005 Galectin-3 expression in parathyroid carcinoma: immunohistochemical study of 26 cases. *Hum. Pathol*. 36:908-914.

[75] Haven CJ, van Puijenbroek M, Karperien M, Fleuren GJ, Morreau H 2004 Differential expression of the calcium sensing receptor and combined loss of chromosomes 1q and 11q in parathyroid carcinoma. *J. Pathol*. 202:86-94.

[76] Cetani F, Picone A, Cerrai P, Vignali E, Borsari S, Pardi E, Viacava P, Naccarato AG, Miccoli P, Kifor O, Brown EM, Pinchera A, Marcocci C 2000 Parathyroid expression of calcium-sensing receptor protein and in vivo parathyroid hormone Ca2+ set point in patients with primary hyperparathyroidism. *J. Clin. Endocrinol. Metab*. 85: 4789-94.

[77] Tan MH, Morrison C, Wang P, Yang X, Haven CJ, Zhang C, Zhao P, Tretiakova MS, Korpi-Hyovalti E, Burgess JR, Soo KC, Cheah WK, Cao B, Resau J, Morreau H, Teh BT 2004 Loss of parafibromin immunoreactivity is a distinguishing feature of parathyroid carcinoma. *Clin. Cancer Res.* 10:6629-6637.

[78] Gill AJ, Clarkson A, Gimm O, Keil J, Dralle H, Howell VM, Marsh DJ 2006 Loss of nuclear expression of parafibromin distinguishes parathyroid carcinomas and hyperparathyroidism-jaw tumor (HPT-JT) syndrome-related adenomas from sporadic parathyroid adenomas and hyperplasias. *Am. J. Surg. Pathol.* 30:1140-1149.

[79] Juhlin CC, Villablanca A, Sandelin K, Haglund F, Nordenström J, Forsberg L, Bränström R, Obara T, Arnold A, Larsson C, Höög A 2007 Parafibromin immunoreactivity: its use as an additional diagnostic marker for parathyroid tumor classification. *Endocr. Relat. Cancer,* 14:501-12.

[80] Juhlin C, Larsson C, Yakoleva T, Leibiger I, Leibiger B, Alimov A, Weber G, Höög A, Villablanca A 2006 Loss of parafibromin expression in a subset of parathyroid adenomas. *Endocr. Relat. Cancer,* 13:509-523.

[81] Cetani F, Pardi E, Ambrogini E, Banti C, Viacava P, Borsari S, Bilezikian JP, Pinchera A, Marcocci C 2008 Hyperparathyroidism 2 gene (*HRPT2, CDC73)* and parafibromin studies in two patients with primary hyperparathyroidism and uncertain pathological assessment. *J. Endocrinol. Invest.* 31:900-904.

[82] Howell VM, Gill A, Clarkson A, Nelson AE, Dunne R, Delbridge LW, Robinson BG, Teh BT, Gimm O, Marsh DJ 2009 Accuracy of combined protein gene product 9.5 and parafibromin markers for immunohistochemical diagnosis of parathyroid carcinoma. 94:434-41

[83] Juhlin CC, Nilsson IL, Johansson K, Haglund F, Villablanca A, Höög A, Larsson C. 2010 Parafibromin and APC as screening markers for malignant potential in atypical parathyroid adenomas. Endocr. Pathol. 21:166-77.

[84] Fernandez-Ranvier GG, Jensen K, Khanafshar E, Quivey JM, Glastonbury C, Kebebew E, Duh QY, Clark OH 2007 Nonfunctioning parathyroid carcinoma: case report and review of literature. *Endocr. Pract.* 13:750-757.

[85] Rubin MR, Silverberg SJ, D'Amour P, Brossard JH, Rousseau L, Sliney J Jr, Cantor T, Bilezikian JP 2007 An N-terminal molecular form of parathyroid hormone (PTH) distinct from hPTH(1-84) is overproduced in parathyroid carcinoma. *Clin. Chem.* 53:1470-1476.

[86] Rubin MR, Bilezikian JP, Birken S, Silverberg SJ 2008 Human chorionic gonadotropin measurements in parathyroid carcinoma. *Eur. J. Endocrinol.* 159:469-474.

[87] Wang C, Gaz R 1983 Natural history of parathyroid carcinoma: diagnosis, treatment and results. *Am. J. Surg.* 149:522-527.

[88] Kebebew E 2001 Parathyroid carcinoma. *Curr. Treat Options Oncol.* 2:347-354.

[89] Koea JB, Shaw JH 1999 Parathyroid cancer: biology and management. *Surg. Oncol.* 8:155-165.

[90] Ippolito G, Palazzo FF, Sebag F, De Micco C, Henry JF 2007 Intraoperative diagnosis and treatment of parathyroid cancer and atypical parathyroid adenoma. *Br. J. Surg.* 94:566-570.

[91] J. Kirkby-Bott, P. Lewis, C. Harmer, W.J.B Smellie. *Towards one stage treatment of parathyroid cancer: High pre-operative index of suspicion and use of frozen section. EJSO*, 2005: 31; 78-83.

[92] Holmes EC, Morton DL, Ketcham AS 1969 Parathyroid carcinoma: a collective review. *Ann. Surg.* 169:631-40.

[93] Fernandez-Ranvier GG, Khanafshar E, Jensen K, Zarnegar R, Lee J, Kebebew E, Duh QY, Clark OH, Parathyroid Carcinoma, Atypical Parathyroid Adenoma, or Parathyromatosis? *Cancer*. 2007;110:255-64.

[94] Sundelin K, Tullgren O, Farnebo LO 1994 Clinical course of metastatic parathyroid cancer. *World J. Surg.* 18:594-598.

[95] Johnston LB, Carroll MJ, Britton KE, Lowe DG, Shand W, Besser GM, Grossman AB 1996 The accuracy of parathyroid gland localization in primary hyperparathyroidism using sestamibi radionuclide imaging. *J. Clin. Endocrinol. Metab.* 81:346-52.

[96] Martinez DA, King DR, Romshe C, Lozano RA, Morris JD, O'Dorisio MS, Martin E Jr 1995 Intraoperative identification of parathyroid gland pathology: a new approach. *J. Pediatr. Surg.* 30:1306-09.

[97] Marcocci C, Mazzeo S, Bruno-Bossio G, Picone A, Vignali E, Ciampi M, Viacava P, Naccarato AG, Miccoli P, Iacconi P, Pinchera A 1998 Preoperative localization of suspicious parathyroid adenomas by assay of parathyroid hormone in needle aspirates. *Eur. J. Endocrinol.* 139:72-77.

[98] Spinelli C, Bonadio AG, Berti P, Materazzi G, Miccoli P 2000 Cutaneous spreading of parathyroid carcinoma after fine needle aspiration cytology. *J. Endocrinol. Invest.* 23:255-257.

[99] Anderson B, Samaan N, Vassilopoulou-Sellin R, Ordonez N, Hickey R 1983 Parathyroid carcinoma: features and difficulties in diagnosis and management. *Surgery,* 94:906-915.

[100] Wynne A, Heerden JV, Carney J, Fitzpatrick L 1992 Parathyroid carcinoma: Clinical and pathological features in 43 patients. *Medicine* 71:197-205.

[101] Rao SR, Shaha AR, Singh B, Rinaldo A, Ferito A 2002 Management of cancer of the parathyroid. *Acta Otolaryngol.* 122:448-452.

[102] Munson ND, Foote RL, Northcutt RC, Tiegs RD, Fitzpatrick LA, Grant CS, van Heerden JA, Thompson GB, Lloyd RV 2003 Parathyroid carcinoma: is there a role for adjuvant radiation therapy? *Cancer* 98:2378-2384.

[103] J. Kirkby-Bott, P. Lewis, C. Harmer, W.J.B Smellie. Towards one stage treatment of parathyroid cancer: High pre-operative index of suspicion and use of frozen section. *EJSO* 2005: 31; 78-83.

[104] Busaidy NL, Jimenez C, Habra MA, Schultz PN, El-Naggar AK, Clayman GL, Asper JA, Diaz EM Jr, Evans DB, Gagel RF, Garden A, Hoff AO, Lee JE, Morrison WH, Rosenthal DI, Sherman SI, Sturgis EM, Waguespack SG, Weber RS, Wirfel K, Vassilopoulou-Sellin R 2004 Parathyroid carcinoma: a 22-year experience. *Head Neck,* 26:716-726.

[105] Clayman GL, Gonzalez HE, El-Naggar A, Vassilopoulou-Sellin R 2004 Parathyroid carcinoma: evaluation and interdisciplinary management. *Cancer* 100:900-905.

[106] Denney AM, Watts NB 2004 The effect of octreotide on parathyroid carcinoma. *J. Clin. Endocrinol. Metab.* 89:1016.

[107] Nemeth EF, Steffey ME, Hammerland LG, Hung BC, Van Wagenen BC, DelMar EG, Balandrin MF 1998 Calcimimetics with potent and selective activity on the parathyroid calcium receptor. *Proc. Natl. Acad. Sci. U S A,* 95:4040-4045.

[108] Collins MT, Skarulis MC, Bilezikian JP, Silverberg SJ, Spiegel AM, Marx SJ 1998 Treatment of hypercalcemia secondary to parathyroid carcinoma with a novel calcimimetic agent. *J. Clin. Endocrinol. Metab.* 93:1083-1088.

[109] Silverberg SJ, Rubin MR, Faiman C, Peacock M, Shoback DM, Smallridge RC, Schwanauer LE, Olson KA, Klassen P, Bilezikian JP 2007 Cinacalcet hydrochloride reduces the serum calcium concentration in inoperable parathyroid carcinoma. *J. Clin. Endocrinol. Metab.* 92:3803-3808.

[110] Marcocci C, Chanson P, Shoback D, Bilezikian J, Fernandez-Cruz L, Orgiazzi J, Henzen C, Cheng S, Sterling LR, Lu J, Peacock M 2009 Cinacalcet reduces serum calcium concentrations in patients with intractable primary hyperparathyroidism. *J. Clin. Endocrinol. Metab.* 94:2766-2772.

[111] Bradwell AR, Harvey TC 1999 Control of hypercalcaemia of parathyroid carcinoma by immunisation. *Lancet,* 353:370-373.

[112] Betea D, Bradwell AR, Harvey TC, Mead GP, Schmidt-Gayk H, Ghaye B, Daly AF, Beckers A 2004 Hormonal and biochemical normalization and tumor shrinkage induced by anti-parathyroid hormone immunotherapy in a patient with metastatic parathyroid carcinoma. *J. Clin. Endocrinol. Metab.* 89:3413-3420.

[113] Shoback DM, Arends RH, Roskos L, Shetty S, Wyres M, Huang S, Raienbell GM 2004 Treatment of parathyroid carcinoma with ABX10241, a monoclonal antibody to parathyroid hormone. *J. Bone Min. Res.* 17 SA498 (abstract).

[114] Schott M, Feldkamp J, Schattenberg D, Krueger T, Dotzenrath C, Seissler J, Scherbaum WA 2000 Induction of cellular immunity in a parathyroid carcinoma treated with tumor lysate-pulsed dendritic cells. *Eur. J. Endocrinol.* 142:300-306.

In: Parathyroid: Anatomy, Functions and Disorders
Editor: James Kirkby-Bott
ISBN: 978-1-62100-765-4

Chapter VIII

Primary Hyperparathyroidism-Diagnosis and Management

James Kirkby-Bott
Kingston Hospital, Surrey, UK

Abstract

Primary hyperparathyroidism is an uncommon clinical entity with a variable worldwide incidence. The incidence and mode of presentation has changed with advances in biochemical assays. Most patients in the West now present earlier diagnosed on biochemical assay results rather than gross physical signs and radiology changes. Neuro-psychiatric symptoms with their insidious onset have become the most common presenting complaint. The development of intact PTH assays and quick PTH assays as well as ultrasound, Sestamibi and most recently 4D triphasic CT scanning has altered the surgical approach and improved surgical outcomes so that 95% of patients are cured at surgery.

Introduction

Primary hyperparathyroidism is an uncommon clinical entity with a variable worldwide incidence. The incidence and mode of presentation has changed with advances in biochemical assays and greater knowledge of the role of parathyroid hormone and its interaction with vitamin D. Most patients in the West now present earlier diagnosed on biochemical assay results rather than gross physical signs and radiology changes. This chapter focuses on how pHPT presents, diagnostic pitfalls and the use of intra-operative adjuncts.

Incidence

Primary hyperparathyroidism (pHPT) is an uncommon clinical entity with wide geographical variation in incidence. In the US it affects 43/100,000[1]. In southern Europe it affects 30/100,000[2]. It is more frequent in women than men but the incidence increases with age in both sexes affecting as many as 210/100,000 55-75 year old women [2]. The technological advances in biochemical assays have also had a large affect on incidence as diagnosis shifts from gross physical symptoms prior to the calcium assays introduced in the 1970s towards asymptomatic detection on routine screening for medical illnesses and earlier presentation with milder symptoms. This may be reflected in the earlist reports of parathyroid surgery in the 1920s and 1930s on patients that probably had parathyroid cancers [3], which reflects the experimental nature of parathyroid surgery at that time, with the grossest cases being operated upon. A reported incidence as low as 10/100,000 in 1980s in the US [4]. The effect of the introduction of the automated calcium analyser is shown by the fivefold increase in incidence of pHPT in the US in the 1970s followed by a decreased incidence during the 1980s as the impact of the 'catch up phenomena' wore off [1]. The incidence of pHPT is also affected by region under study, nutritional status of the studied population, provision of healthcare and availability of biochemical screening. Irradiation of the neck is also strongly associated with the development of pHPT [5].

Clinical Presentation

As diagnosis and presentation occurs earlier in the disease fewer patients present with the grossest symptoms of pHPT. Classically the symptoms of hypercalcaemia were described as "Bones, stones, abdominal groans and psychic moans. Representing Osteomalacia and osteoporosis, renal calculi, Constipation and anxiety, confusion and depression. The full list of symptoms and signs can be found in table 1. Such presenting manifestations are rare in the West today, but nephrolithiasis and hypertension (due to direct arterial and myocardial effects rather than just renal impairment) are still the most commonly cited preoperative conditions, but controlled studies of presenting symptoms show that up to 80% of patients present with nonspecific symptoms of depression, lethargy and fatigue. As they come on insidiously, onset of symptoms is often not fully recognised by patients pre-operatively [6]. Symptoms can be related either to hypercalcemia or elevated PTH independent of the hypercalcaemia.

Diagnosis

Hypercalcaemia in the setting of elevated PTH levels is usually diagnostic of pHPT as in malignant hypercalcaemia the PTH level is normal or suppressed which is the appropriate response in hypercalcaemia due to causes other than pHPT. 25 OH vitamin D deficiency can also make diagnosis difficult as mild pHPT has the calcium levels suppressed by the low vitamin D levels. Correction of vitamin D in such patients results in hypercalcaemia with continued elevation of PTH levels compared to secondary HPT due to vitamin D deficiency when correction of vitamin D levels doesn't produce hypercalcaemia and the PTH levels return towards normal. Additionally low phosphate levels are seen in pHPT. Final confirmation can be made by measuring the urine/plasma calcium:creatinine clearance ratio. This requires 24hr urine collection for calcium and creatinine paired with a serum calcium and creatinine level during the urine collection period (fig 1).

The calcium:creatinine clearance ratio allows one to differentiate familial hypercalcaemic hypocalciuria(FHH) from pHPT. FHH presents with high calcium and PTH levels but reduced urine excretion and doesn't respond to parathyroid resection at surgery it is discussed in detail in chapter 5 on familial pHPT. A calcium creatinine clearance ratio of <0.01 is diagnostic of FHH whereas a level of >0.01 (or in some texts 0.02) [6] is suggestive of pHPT. However, vitamin D deficiency artificially lowers the calcium: creatinine clearance ratio so needs to be corrected where equivocal results up to 0.02 are found[7]. Lithium causes elevated calcium and PTH levels through alterations in the set-point of calcium sensing receptors. However, urinary calcium is not elevated in lithium induced parathyroid hyperplasia and bone mineral density is not affected either [8]. Despite this a small number of patients on lithium do present with localisable disease and are cured by focused parathyroidectomy [9]. It is uncertain if this represents a sub group of patients that develop adenomatous disease whilst on lithium rather than hyperplasia, but of 1207 surgical pHPT operations 1.3% were taking lithium beforehand [10] equivalent to a 130/100,000 population incidence. Significantly more than the general population. Lithium induced hyperplasia however doesn't require surgery whereas adenomatous disease does [7].

Table 1. Symptoms of pHPT. Most are related to hypercalcaemia but some are independent of calcium and due to elevated PTH levels

Organ System	Symptoms
GI tract	Nausea/vomiting, Pancreatitis, Peptic ulcer disease, Anorexia, Weight loss, Constipation
Cardiovascular	Hypertension, Bradycardia, Atrial fibrillation/flutter, heart block
Renal	Renal stones, Polyuria, Thirst and polydipsia, Renal impairment due to nephrocalcinosis and or pre-renal failure
Neuro-cognitive	Anxiety, Headaches, Confusion, paranoia, Depression, Ataxia, Coma
Musculo-skeletal	Muscle weakness, myalgia, bone pain, osteomalacia and osteoporosis
Miscellaneous	Visual disturbance, Band keratopathy, Conjunctivitis, Pruritis

$$\frac{(\text{urine calcium (mmol/l) x plasma creatinine } (\mu\text{mol/l}) \text{ /1000})}{(\text{plasma calcium (mmol/l) x urine creatinine (mmol/l)})}$$

Figure 1. Formula for measuring calcium:creatinine ratio. To convert mg/dl to mmol/l multiply by 0.25.

Intra-Operative Adjuncts to Parathyroid Surgery

Changing biochemical assay availability and reliability has altered the surgical strategies used in parathyroid surgery. The conventional operation was a bilateral neck exploration which involved searching both sides, identifying all 4 parathyroid glands and removing the one that looked most like an adenoma. Of 6331 cases of non familial pHPT 87% were found to have single adenomas, 9% had four-gland hyperplasia and 3% had multiple adenomas[11].

Fewer than 1% had carcinoma [12]. Given these findings, which are not disputed, is bilateral exploration required when 97% can be diagnosed with a unilateral exploration? George Irvin in Miami, developed the use of intra-operative PTH (IOPTH) measurements in the 1990s to confirm surgical cure after focused parathyroidectomy, allowing parathyroidectomy to become an outpatient procedure for many[13,14].

Advances in the sensitivity and specificity of ultrasound and then combined with the use of Sestamibi led to patients with concordant imaging results having similar cure rates to parathyroidectomy with IOPTH after focused parathyroidectomy without IOPTH measurement[15,16].

In the 3rd ESES workshop review paper on intra-operative adjuncts it was suggested that IOPTH should be used only with Sestamibi localised disease and not in concordant USS and Sestamibi localisation where it was of no proven benefit[17]. Many other techniques have been used to help surgeons localise parathyroid tissue at surgery including frozen section and intra-operative tisue aspirates. IV methylene blue dye and radioguided parathyroidectomy. All of these are compared in the 3rd ESES workshop paper by Harrison in 2009. Table 2 compares techniques. Radioguided parathyroidectomy works similarly to sentinel node biopsy.

A radioactive tracer is injected into the patient and adenoma localised by gamma radiation levels from the affected gland. Methylene blue is associated with a low risk of encephalopathic toxicity and is not recommended. Intra-operative tissue aspiration has a 100% specificity and normal and diseased glands produce significantly different levels [18,19,20,21] it is particularly useful in concomitant thyroid nodular disease that can make parathyroid localisation more difficult.

Table 2. Comparison of intra-operative adjuncts

Intra-operative adjunct	Level of evidence	Additional notes
Radioguided parathyroidectomy	Level IV	Requires a positive preopertive Sestamibi scan
Frozen section	Level III-IV	Microscopic follicular variants can cause false negatives and positives.
Methylene Blue	Level IV	Risk of toxic encephalopathy particularly if taking an SSRI drug
Tissue aspirate PTH	Level IIb	Validated in pHPT

Decision to Operate

As in all surgeries this is a multi-factorial decision. There is evidence that age should not be a barrier as elderly patients potentially have a lot to gain as improvements in musculoskeletal pain, improved bone densitometry, amelioration of insidious neuro-cognitive symptoms and a reduced number of medications can all be outcomes seen after successful parathyroidectomy that may lead to an increase in patients quality of life. [22] [23] [24] [25].

Local anaesthesia is feasible in open minimally invasive approaches especially when combined with sedation rather than full general anaesthesia so that most co-mordities need to be contra-indications to parathyroidectomy. The surgical approach depends upon the localization results and figure 8.2 suggests an algorithm for this. Chapter 9 gives detailed review of the currently used surgical approaches in primary HPT.

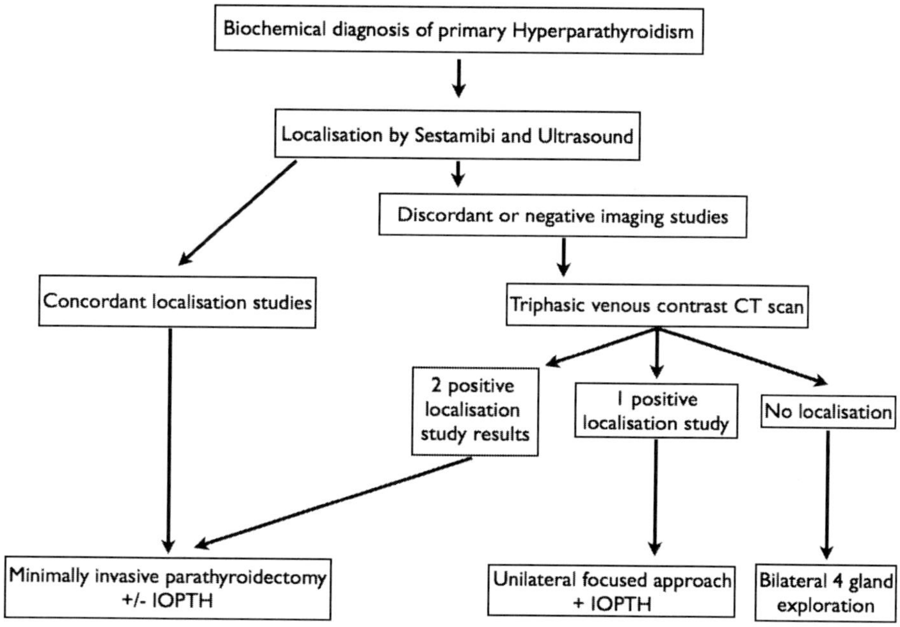

Figure 8.2. Suggested algorithm for deciding on the surgical approach used in pHPT.

Conclusion

The incidence of pHPT is increasing with increased awareness and use of biochemical screening. Knowledge of the pathophysiology of parathyroid glands and presentation of parathyroid disease aids diagnosis and improved localisation has revolutionised the surgical approach. IOPTH is useful in certain situations as are intra-operative adjuncts, particularly parathyroid tissue aspirates in concomitant thyroid disease. However, the best localisation technique remains 'the localisation of an experienced parathyroid surgeon.'

References

[1] Melton JL. The epidemiology of primary hyperparathyroidism in North America. *J. Bone Miner. Res.* 2002; 17(Suppl 2):N12-17.

[2] Adami S, Marcocci C, Gatti D. Epidemiology of primary hyperparathyroidsim in Europe. *J. Bone Miner. Res.* 2002; 17(Suppl 2):N18-23.

[3] Lew JI, Solorzano CC. Surgical Management of Primary Hyperparathyroidism: State of the Art. In Surgical Clinics of North America: Endocrine Surgery, Zeiger MA editor. 2009; 89(5). Saunders, Philadelphia.

[4] Heath HW III, Hodgson SF, Kennedy MA. Primary hyperparathyroidism: incidence, morbidity and potential economic impact on the community. *N. Eng. J. Med.* 1980; 302:189-93.

[5] Christensson T. Hyperparathyroidism and radiation therapy. *Ann. Intern Med.* 1978;89:216-7.

[6] Belezikan JP, Potts JP. Asymptomatic primary hyperparathyroidism: new issues and questions. *J. Bone Miner. Res.* 2002; 17 (Suppl 2):N57-67.

[7] Kirkby-Bott J, El-Khatib Z. Recent advances in parathyroid surgery. In Johnson CD (editor), Recent advances in surgery vol 33.2010; Jaypee Brothers Medical Publishers, Delhi.

[8] Zamani A, Omrani GR, Nasab MM. Lithium's effect on bone mineral density. *Bone* 2009;44:331-4.

[9] Carchman E, Ogilvie J, Holst J, Yim J, Carty S. Appropriate surgical treatment of lithium-associated HPT. *World J. Surg.* 2008;32:2195-9.

[10] Hundley JC, Woodrum DT, Saunders BD, Doherty GM, Gauger PG. Revisiting lithium-associated HPT in the era of intraoperative parathyroid hormone monitoring. *Surgery* 2005; 138:1027-31.

[11] Davies M, Fraser WD, Hosking DJ. The management of primary hyperparathyroidism. *Clinical Endocrinology* 2002; 57:145-155.

[12] Denham DW, Norman J. Cost-effectiveness of preoperative sestamibi scan for primary hyperparathyroidism is dependent solely upon the surgeon's choice of operative procedure. *J. Am. Coll. Surg.* 1998;186:293-305.

[13] Irvin GL, Prudhomme DL, Deriso GT, et al. A new approach to parathyroidectomy. *Ann. Surg.* 1994;219:574-81.

[14] Irvin GL, Sfakianakis G, Yeung L, et al. Ambulatory parathyroidectomy for primary hyperparathyroidism. *Arch. Surg.* 1996; 131:1074-8.

[15] Suliburk JW, Sywak MS, Sidhu SB, Delbridge LW. 1000 minimally invasive parathyroidectomies without intra-operative parathyroid hormone measurement: Lessons learnt. *ANZ J. Surg.* 2011;81:362-5.

[16] Stalberg P, Sidhu S, Sywak M, Robinson B, Wilinson M, Delbridge L. Intraoperaive parathyroid measurement during minimally invasive parathyroidectomy: Does it "value -add" to decision-making? *J. Am. Coll. Surg.* 2006;203:1-6.

[17] Harrison BJ, Triponez F. Intraoperative adjuncts in surgery for primary HPT. *Langenbecks Arch. Surg.* 2009;394:799-809.

[18] Kirkby-Bott J, Carnaille B. Experience of the reliability of intra-operative sampling of tissue PTH in parathyroid surgery (letter to the editor). *World J. Surg.* (2010) 34:2254.

[19] Chan RK, Ibrahim SI, Pil P, Tanasijevic M, Moore F. Validation of amethod to replace frozen sectionduring parathyroid exploration by using the rapid parathyroid hormone assay on parathyroid aspirates. *Arch. Surg.* 2005;140:371-3.

[20] Perrier ND, Ituarte P, Kikuchi S, Siperstein AE, Duh QY, Clark OH, et al. Intraoperative parathyroid aspiration and parathyroid hormone assay as an alternative to frozen section for tissue identification. *World J. Surg.* 2000;24:1319-22.

[21] Horányi J, Duffek L, Szlávik R et al (2010) Intraoperative determination of PTH concentrations in fine needle tissue aspirates to identify parathyroid tissue during parathyroidectomy. *World J. Surg.* 34:538–543.

[22] Bachar G, Gilat H, Mizrachi A, et al. Comparison of perioperative management and outcome of parathyroidectomy between older and younger patients. *Head Neck* 2008; 30(11):1415-21.

[23] Egan KR, Adler JT, Olson JE, Chen H. Parathyroidectomy for primary hyperparathyroidism in octogenarians and nonagenarians: a risk-benefit analysis. *J Surg Res* 2007; 140(2):194-8.

[24] Uden P, Chan A, Duh QY, et al. Primary hyperparathyroidism in younger and older patients: symptoms and outcome of surgery. *World J Surg* 1992; 16(4):791-7; discussion 798.

[25] Stechman MJ, Weisters M, Gleeson FV, et al. Parathyroidectomy is safe and improves symptoms in elderly patients with PHPT. *Clin Endocrinol (Oxf)* 2009.

Part 4:
Treatment of Parathyroid Disorder

In: Parathyroid: Anatomy, Functions and Disorders
Editor: James Kirkby-Bott
ISBN: 978-1-62100-765-4

Chapter IX

Surgery for Primary Hyperparathyroidism

Ziad El-Khatib and Hiba El Hage Chehade
Makassed General Hospital, Beirut, Lebanon

Abstract

Advances in the accuracy of preoperative and peri-operative localizing techniques has lead to a preference for a minimally invasive procedure over bilateral exploration in image localized sporadic primary hyperparathyroidism. The focused approach has been shown to be equivalent to bilateral exploration for cure rate and superior to it concerning cosmetic result, duration of the intervention, postoperative stay, and hypocalcaemia, as assessed by prospective and randomized trials. [61,62]. During the last decade, multiple minimally invasive approaches have been described [63], including: minimally invasive open parathyroidectomy, endoscopic and video-assisted parathyroidectomy and extra-cervical access from incisions in the chest wall and/or axilla.

The first endoscopic parathyroidectomy was described initially by Gagner in 1996. Minimally invasive video-assisted parathyroidectomy was first described by Miccoli et al. [47], and totally endoscopic parathyroidectomy by the lateral approach by Henry et al. [13]. Currently the best indication for the latter approach is adenomas that lie deep to the thyroid lobe, usually arising from superior gland adenomas.

All these minimally invasive techniques rely on preoperative localizing studies and may benefit from intra-operative PTH monitoring in certain scenarios as shown by Barczynski et al. [64]. The major problem with endoscopic parathyroidectomy is the limited working space so that associated nodular thyroid disease and the presence of a large (3 cm) parathyroid adenoma are relative contraindications. It has also been difficult to show a real advantage for endoscopic versus open minimally invasive surgery, largely due to the expense of the endoscopic equipment required. In 2006 Barczynski published a prospective, randomized trial on open versus video-assisted techniques [38]. This showed a preference in the minimally invasive video assisted parathyroidectomy (MIVAP) group due to an easier recognition of the recurrent laryngeal nerve, less postoperative pain and a better cosmetic results. On the other hand, there was a significantly higher operative cost. [65]

This chapter will shed the light on these different procedures along with the indications, limitations, and adavantages.

Introduction

Historical Background

The first successful parathyroidectomy was performed by Mandel in 1925. [74] Since then, bilateral parathyroid exploration performed through a transverse cervicotomy has remained the standard procedure. [36,39] In 1975, Roth et al advocated the unilateral exploration. [75] However, the concept of minimally invasive parathyroid surgery emerged in the early 1980s. [36] The pioneering work was proposed by Tibblin et al in 1982, with a unilateral exploration based on finding a single adenoma and an ipsilateral normal gland. [76]

Nowadays, surgical treatment for primary hyperparathyroidism is on the rise worldwide due to several reasons. It causes symptomatic relief, [40] improves cardiovascular status [77] and controls diabetes post-op, [78,79,80] and even leads to a sense of wellness and improved function in asymptomatic patients. [81] Added to these reasons is the introduction of minimally invasive surgery, which is applied in around 50% of the patients. [36]

Because sporadic primary HPT is caused by a solitary parathyroid adenoma in 85-90% of cases, [6,39] usually of small size and high prevalence in women, [36] it represented an attractive field for the application of the minimally invasive approach. The concept of limited exploration was reinforced by the development of improved localization studies such as sestamibi scan and ultrasonography, the introduction of intraoperative quick parathyroid hormone assay, and the introduction of cervicoscopy. [41,66]

Minimally invasive parathyroidectomy (MIP) may be divided into two groups: mini-open approaches performed under direct vision via a small cervical incision and techniques using the endoscope. [36] In addition, several other approaches have been also described: from the chest wall, the breast, and the axilla, which have gained its widest acceptance from the Asian community. [41]

Definition of Minimally Invasive Parathyroidectomy (MIP)

Minimally invasive surgery can be defined as the ability of the surgeon to perform traditional surgical procedures in novel ways to minimize the trauma of the surgical exposure. [83]

The philosophy of minimally invasive surgery does not depend only on the length of the skin incision; it also, and above all, takes into consideration the extent of dissection with preservation of vital structures, and the accessibility of the operative field.

Therefore, MIP should properly be defined as operations through a short, less than 3 cm, [36,82] discrete cervical incision that permits direct access to the thyroid or parathyroid gland, resulting in a focused dissection.

In addition, any effort to minimize invasiveness should also take into account the type of anesthesia. Local or regional anesthesia and hypnosedation are two alternatives to general anesthesia because they avoid the complications of the latter. [36]

Indications

Because MIP is a focused technique, it is best proposed for patients with sporadic primary hyperparathyroidism in whom a single adenoma has been clearly localized by preoperative imaging studies. [6,36,41,46] Other factors that are usually taken into consideration are small-sized adenoma (less than 3 cm, to avoid its rupture [41]) and the absence of: previous conventional neck surgery or irradiation, [6,41,46] persistent or recurrent hyperparathyroidism, mediastinal adenoma, suspicion of multiple gland disease such as MEN and familial hyperparathyroidism, [41] suspicion of parathyroid malignancy, and concomitant thyroid disease such as a large multinodular goiter or thyroiditis. [6] Depending on the operator's experience and according to the specific technique utilized, these limitations can become relative. [41,46] For instance, endoscopic parathyroidectomy by the lateral approach can be performed in patients who have previously undergone a contralateral neck operation or tracheostomy. [46] There is level V evidence that video-assisted techniques are feasible in cases of secondary hyperparathyroidism and familial primary hyperparathyroidism. There is a grade C recommendation to perform MIVAP in the case of four-gland hyperplasia[41]. However, the scarcity of data suggests the need for controlled, randomized trials to clarify the safety in terms of cure and complication rate of this procedure in comparison with central bilateral neck exploration (CBNE). [41]

Choice of Technique Depending on Gland Position

In 2008, Henry et al suggested a classification system based on three different positions of enlarged parathyroid glands. Position 1 is posterior to the two superior thirds of the posterior surface of the thyroid lobe. These adenomas were supposed to correspond to superior glands. Position 2 is at the level of or below the inferior pole of the thyroid lobe but in a plane posterior to it. These adenomas may be a superior or an inferior gland that has fallen posteriorly and more or less inferiorly into the tracheoesophageal groove. Position 3 is at the level of or below the tip of the inferior pole of the thyroid lobe but in the same plane, that is in a superficial plane. These adenomas, corresponding to inferior glands, can be found in close contact with the inferior pole of the thyroid lobe but also along the thyrothymic ligament or into the superior pole of the thymus. Adenomas in positions 1 and 2 are considered to be located in the vicinity of the recurrent laryngeal nerve, and the endoscopic lateral approach might be more convenient. Adenomas in position 3 are considered to be at a distance from the nerve, which runs more posteriorly; hence, an open minimally invasive parathyroidectomy (oMIP) is considered more suitable. [42] However, different MIP techniques have been proposed and used for any of the aforementioned parathyroid positions. [66]

Choice of Anesthesia

MIP can be performed under general anesthesia. [59] It can also be done under local/regional anesthesia on an ambulatory basis as an effort to minimize the invasiveness of the procedure. [36] Regional anesthesia avoids vocal cord changes seen in up to 5% of patients undergoing endotracheal intubation. [59,84,85]

Furthermore, exploring a conscious patient permits intraoperative assessment of the superior and recurrent laryngeal nerve functions because the patient can vocalize throughout the procedure. [59]

Other advantages of local/regional anesthesia include: decreased operating time, lower incidence of postop nausea and vomiting, lower postoperative pain, shorter recovery period, and less cost. [59,84]

In theory, selective parathyroidectomy (SP) under local/regional anesthesia may be beneficial for older patients with severe comorbidities. Major concerns include a slight increase in risk the of postoperative bleeding and hematoma formation [59], particularly when local anaesthetic with adrenaline is used.

Open Minimally Invasive Parathyroidectomy (oMIP)

It is the most frequently performed MIP, and it is associated with more than 97% success rate even without the use of iPTH. [40]

The operation is carried out under general or regional anaesthesia with sedation. A 2-3cm incision is made 2cm above the sternal notch. [36,38] The platysma muscle is divided in the line of the incision. The anterior border of the sternocleidomastoid muscle (SCM) is then identified and freed in both cranial and caudal directions. The space between the SCM and the carotid sheath structures laterally and the strap muscles medially is opened. The lateral lobe of the thyroid gland is identified and, if necessary, delivered into the wound. A careful search is then made for the parathyroid tumour, which is identified, mobilised and removed after securing its vascular pedicle using small vascular clips. The thyroid lobe is then replaced, drains are not routinely used. The wound is closed with an absorbable subcuticular sutures. [37]

This procedure is a safe, [38,39] cost effective technique allowing treatment of primary hyperparathyroidism on an ambulatory basis. It has a cure rate comparable to conventional surgery. [39] However, surgical exploration is limited and hindered by the length of the skin incision: the shorter the skin incision, the more difficult the oMIP. This is particularly true for deep-seated parathyroid adenomas in patients with large and short necks. [36]

Minimally Invasive Video-Assisted Parathyroidectomy (MIVAP)

Minimally invasive video-assisted parathyroidectomy (MIVAP) was first described by Miccoli et al in 1998. [73,86] Early after its first description, this technique encountered a large worldwide spread. The procedure is done under general or locoregional anesthesia with a bilateral superficial cervical block. The patient is placed in the supine position, without hyperextension of the neck, so as to increase the working space under the strap muscles.

The skin is prepared to allow a possible conversion to the traditional cervicotomy. A 15mm transverse incision is performed 2 cm above the sternal notch, subcutaneous fat and platysma are carefully dissected. The cervical linea alba is divided longitudinally for up to 4 cm. [47,51] At the beginning of the experience, the procedure implied a short CO_2

insufflation to facilitate dissection of the thyroid lobe from the strap muscles [41,53]. After a short initial experience, the procedure was changed in a completely gasless approach.

The strap muscles on the side of the adenoma are then gently retracted with one small conventional retractor. A second retractor is placed directly on the thyroid lobe, which is retracted medially and lifted up. The dissection of the lobe from the strap muscles is performed under direct vision. A 5mm 30 degree endoscope, is then introduced through the incision. Needlescopic surgical instruments are used.

The procedure is then conducted endoscopically. Three surgeons are needed to perform the video assisted procedure. The operator holds a spatula for dissection. The first assistant holds the endoscope and a spatula-aspirator. The second assistant holds the small retractors. The first step of the endoscopic stage of the procedure consists of completing the liberation of the thyroid gland from the strap muscles to have a good exposure of the parathyroid sites. Endoscopic dissection comprises division of the middle thyroid vein, either between 5mm vascular clips or with the harmonic scalpel.

The operative field is then completely exposed, with the carotid artery laterally, vertebral plane posteriously and thyro-tracheal groove medially. Exploration can start using small atraumatic spatulas. The exploration starts on the side in which the adenoma is supposed to be on the basis of the preoperative imaging.

The magnification (twofold to threefold) of the endoscope permits an easy identification of the nerve and the parathyroid glands, if the principles of blunt and bloodless dissection are respected. The use of monopolar cautery or harmonic scalpel is postponed until the recurrent laryngeal nerve, that generally lies near the parathyroid gland, is visualized. Once the adenoma is located, gentle and accurate manipulation is mandatory. When the hylus of the parathyroid gland is reached, and completely dissected, the vessels are ligated. The adenoma is removed and retrieved through the incision. After checking the hemostasis, the strap muscles are sutured along the midline as well as the platysma.

The skin is closed by means of an absorbable subcuticular running suture and/or by a skin sealant. No drainage is required. [47,48,51,45,49,6] The advantage of MIVAP is the feasibility of bilateral neck exploration. [45,49,66] This is important whenever there is a suspicion of multiglandular disease. This has led to initiation of further studies to evaluate the efficacy and rationale of video-assisted parathyroidectomy compared to conventional bilateral exploration for parathyroidectomy in secondary HPT patients. Bilateral neck exploration in MIVAP also makes equivocal pre-op localization studies only a relative exclusion criterion for this MIP approach.

It can also allow concomitant thyroid resection in selected cases further reducing the exclusion criteria and conversion rate with respect to the lateral approach. The main technical limitation for MIVAP is the adenoma size (extraction of large adenomas through a small incision can lead to rupture of the parathyroid capsule, [41] hence, possibly leading to parathyromatosis). The conversion rate is around 8% [47] and it could appear high particularly if comparing it to that of video-assisted thyroidectomy; the reasons for conversion though are often linked with the specific problems of PHPT, including negative explorations or intrathyroid lesions, rather than with technical pitfalls. [47,6,41]

Some authors proposed MIVAP variants. In 2001, Lorenz et al. [54,87] illustrated a modified MIVAP using a separate 5-mm incision caudal to the main access, harboring a newly designed self-cutting, bland trocar with an additional gas insufflation port. A 5 mm 30 degree magnifying endoscopic camera is introduced and continuous gas insufflation during the open phase of preparation serves as a coagulation smoke radiator to prevent obscured vision and interference with the preparation, thus guaranteeing free and full range camera sight.

The recurrent laryngeal nerve is routinely identified and monitored with neurostimulation. Optical identification of the refined cervical structures is amplified by videoscopic magnification. [54,41] Other authors suggested combining two mini-invasive procedures, performing radioguided video-assisted parathyroidectomy to exploit the advantages of both techniques. [55,56]

Endoscopic Parathyroidectomy

Anterior Cervical Approach

Complete endoscopic parathyroidectomy by an anterior approach was first described by Gagner in 1996. [1,12]

Under general anesthesia, the patient is placed in a supine position with his neck in minimal extension. The neck area is prepared and draped in the fashion typical for conventional surgery. A 5-mm skin incision is made just above the sternal notch in the lower midline of the neck. One sharply dissects until below the platysma. Then, a 5-mm trocar is inserted. A purse-string suture, picking up the platysma layer and investing fascia, is placed around the trocar, to create an air-tight seal. Afterwards, carbon dioxide is insufflated to 10mmHg. A 5 mm zero-degree endoscope is inserted through the trocar, and the subplatysmal tissue is very gently bluntly dissected with the tip of the telescope to develop the avascular subplatysmal space. Dissection of this plane is concentrated on the side of the localized adenoma. Once enough space has been created, a 30-degree endoscope is used for the remainder of the case. Another 5-mm port is placed in the ipsilateral neck about 2 to 3 cm anterior to the sternocleidomastoid muscle. An endoscopic scissors is used for additional blunt and sharp dissection to enlarge the subplatysmal space. A working area of approximately 5 × 7 cm is formed. Two additional 5-mm ports are placed for the procedure, one in the ipsilateral neck and another in the contralateral neck. Using an endoscopic hook and an electrocautery, the strap muscles are divided at midline and retracted laterally. The thyroid lobe is mobilized anteromedially to allow for visualization of the ipsilateral parathyroid glands. If deemed necessary for this purpose, the middle thyroid vein is isolated, clipped, and divided. The parathyroid adenoma is usually visualized when the fascia connecting the thyroid lobe with the carotid sheath is divided. The recurrent laryngeal nerve is identified in all cases. The vascular pedicle of the adenoma is dissected and divided using small clips. The gland is then removed via the 5mm trocar site. Bilateral exploration might be carried out via the symmetrically placed trocars to compare the rest of the glands with the extracted one. Some surgeons recommend that the ipsilateral parathyroid gland be identified; identification of this gland in conjunction with intraoperative PTH monitoring helps exclude the possibility of parathyroid hyperplasia. The platysma and skin are closed with 4-0 sutures. [1,2,4,5,6,12,41]

A modified technique has been described by Cougard et al in 1997, [7,8] using a 0 degree 5-mm endoscope and an additional two 3-mm trocars inserted laterally to perform a bilateral exploration in cases of multiple gland disease. Under general anesthesia, the neck is in minimal extension. A 1.5 cm midline incision is made just above the suprasternal notch, along the line of the classical cervicotomy. The strap muscles are dissected vertically in the midline. A tip of a scissors is used to separate the superficial and deep muscular planes below the hyoid bone. A 5 mm trocar is inserted and fixed with a purse string suture. CO2 insufflation is started at a rate of 1 l/min to a maximum of 8mmHg. A 5 mm 0° endoscope is inserted. Its tip is used to create a working space between the avascular intermusclar space. Under endoscopic vision, two 3 mm trocars are inserted at each side of the midline. The sites of insertion are chosen after transillumination by the endoscope to avoid the anterior jugular veins. Bilateral neck exploration and dissection of the tissues surrounding the thyroid proceeds. For completion of the exploration, the middle thyroid vein is isolated, clipped or cauterized, and divided if necessary. All four glands are searched for; the adenoma is identified, dissected, resected, and extracted through the midline incision. Hemostasis is secured. Then, closure is performed in layers. [5,6,7,8]

In 1998, a similar technique was reported by Yeung et al, [11] using one 11-mm port in the suprasternal notch and another two 5-mm ports on either side above the lower insertion of the sternocleidomastoid (SCM). The patient is placed in a supine position with his neck in neutral position, under general anesthesia. The neck area is prepared and draped in the fashion typical for conventional surgery. A 11-mm skin incision is made just above the sternal notch in the lower midline of the neck. With the skin edges elevated, a plane is developed deep to the investing fascia of the neck between the anterior borders of the sternocleidomastoid muscles. Carbon dioxide insufflation to 10-15 mmHg (which is then further decreased to 5-8 mmHg after the space is developed) is started underneath the investing fascia of the neck to produce the initial surgical emphysema. A purse-string suture, picking up the platysma layer and investing fascia, is placed around the trocar to prevent both gas leakage and the trocar from slipping out of the wound. A 5-mm trocar is inserted at the medial border of the sternocleidomastoid muscle at a convenient level above the first incision (usually 2-3 cm above that). Sharp dissection is then carried out in this bloodless plane to ensure a working space. To ensure unimpeded movement of adjacent trocars, less bulky trocars are preferred. Plastic cannulas have added advantage of not interfering with cautery. The sternomastoid muscle, nicely enveloped by the the investing fascia of the neck, is part of the roof of the cavity, and should not obscure the dissection. Some bridging veins may need clipping or, better, can be subjected to diathermy. Another 5 mm cannula is then inserted to allow a two-handed technique. The rest of the operation is identical to other techniques. [6, 11]

In 2001, a gasless endoscopic technique was described by Usui et al who use a special retractor and Kirschner wires as lifting devices. [9] Under general anesthesia, the patient is placed in a supine position with the neck hyperextended. A 3–3.5 cm transverse incision is made 2 cm below the clavicle on the side of the tumor. This wound is normally covered with open-neck bandages. Another 0.5-cm incision is made for a 5-mm endoscope on the lateral neck on the side of the tumor. Either a 5-mm laparoscopic grasper or a conventional forceps and an ultrasonically activated scalpel are passed through the transverse incision. After an appropriate dissection of the subplatysmal plane, two pieces of Kirschner wire 1.2 mm in diameter are inserted horizontally into the subcutaneous layer on the anterior neck. These wires are then lifted up and fixed to an L-shaped pole to create the working space. The strap muscles are split longitudinally near the anterior border of the sternocleidomastoid muscle to expose the ipsilateral thyroid gland. A new retractor for both the sternocleidomastoid and the split strap muscles was designed. This retractor consists of a conventional retractor and a shaft. The shaft measures 15 cm long, 1.2mm in diameter, and has a sharpened end to penetrate the skin. The end of this retractor is inserted into the subclavian incision and the shaft penetrates the skin on the outside. As a result, the retractor can be controlled from the outside through a tiny hole, and no additional incision is necessary. The retractor is slightly flattened near the end so that it cannot rotate freely and it is fixed to a special holder. This new retractor creates a sufficient surgical working space, even for the removal of a large tumor. The methods used for thyroid and parathyroid surgery are similar to conventional ones. [9]

Lateral Cervical Approach

Henry et al described an endoscopic technique using a lateral approach along the anterior border of the SCM muscle in 1999. [13] The best indications for endoscopic parathyroidectomy by the lateral approach (EPLA) are adenomas deeply situated in the neck, usually arising from the superior gland; meaning the superior parathyroid glands—as their enlargement pushes them to migrate posteriorly and slide along the prevertebral plane next to the lateral esophageal border; also, for inferior parathyroid glands located posterior to the inferior poles of the thyroid lobe. [14,46] It is in these cases that they become intimate with the recurrent laryngeal nerve. The lateral view permits easy identification of the nerve abutting the adenoma and therefore allows a secure dissection. The lateral approach is not suitable for superficially located parathyroid glands (i.e., the inferior glands located at the lower pole of the thyroid lobe or in the thyrothymic tracts). [46]

Under general anesthesia, the patient is in a supine position without extending the neck to avoid placing much tension on the sternocleidomastoid and strap muscles. Keeping these muscles relaxed and a low insufflation pressure are essential to keep a working place for dissection. [14] The surgeon and his assistant are at the side of the lesion. Three trocars are used: one 10 mm trocar for the 10 mm endoscope for dissection, then 5 mm endoscope for extraction, and two 3 mm trocars. The operator uses several 2.5 mm instruments: scissors, electrocautery, graspers and a blunt dissector rod (Figure 9.1). A 15 mm transversal skin incision is made on the anterior border of the SCM, 3–4 cm above the sternal notch. In the case of conversion to traditional cervicotomy, this incision can be extended. Table 9.1 shows a comparison of trocar placements between aprroached described by Gagner, Henry and Miccoli. After achieving hemostasis in the subcutaneous tissue, the platysma is divided; then, the anterior border of the sternocleidomastoid is freed. Through this incision, the fascia, connecting the posterior portion of the strap muscles and the thyroid lobe to the carotid sheath, is gently divided with scissors, far enough to visualize the prevertebral fascia. The omohyoid muscle forms the superior border of the dissection. The dissection plane is between infrahyoid muscles posteriorly, and the deep surface of the sternocleidomastoid, internal jugular vein, and common carotid artery. Then, the posterior surface of the thyroid is reached.

If needed, the middle thyroid vein can be ligated and divided through this incision. The retrothyroid space maybe further widened by applying a wet gauze against the prevertebral fascia allowing adequate space for the introduction of the endoscope. Two 3 mm trocars are then inserted: the superior one is 4-6cm above the first main incision, and the inferior one is 3-4cm below. The transparietal path of these trocars is made through the incision, from the inside to the outside using a guide stick. The previously inserted wet gauze is removed followed by the introduction of a 10mm trocar through the main incision which is fixed by a purse string including the anterior border of sternocleidomastoid and posterior border of the sternothyroid. This prevents gas leakage and slippage of the trocar. CO2 is insufflated to a pressure of 8mmHg, a pressure sufficient enough to provide a working space and prevent minute bleeding. Unilateral video-assisted parathyroid exploration is then carried out using the 10-mm 0° endoscopic camera. The dissection is performed using 2.5mm instruments. The anatomic structures – posterior aspect of the thyroid lobe, lateral border of the trachea and esophagus, trunk and branches of the inferior thyroid artery, inferior laryngeal nerve and thyrothymic tract – are checked. During this exploration, both the adenoma and the ipsilateral parathyroid gland are identified. The search for the adenoma is always aided by the pre-op localization tests. At this stage, CO2 insufflation is stopped. Figure 9.2 shows trocar positions used. The single midline incision is the access used in Miccoloi's video assited approach. Once the adenoma is dissected, the trocars can be removed.

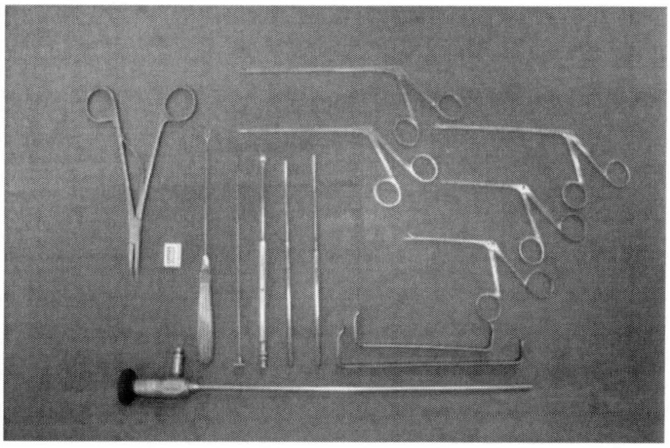

Figure 9.1. Examples of instrumentation set up for Endoscopic and video-assisted parathyroidectomy.

Table 9.1. Comparison of endoscopic techniques

	Endoscopic parathyroidectomy by Gagner	Video-assisted parathyroidectomy by Henry	Minimally invasive video-assisted parathyroidectomy by Miccoli
Number of trocars	3 – 4	3	0
Endoscope diameter	5 mm	10 mm	5 mm
Endoscope angle	Initial 0° then 30°	0°	30°
Other trocars diameter	3 - 5 mm	2.5 mm	-
CO_2 insufflation	10 mmHg	8 mmHg	No
Bilateral approach	No	No	Yes

Then, directly through the skin incision, the thyroid lobe is retracted medially, and the adenoma is extracted, and its pedicle is ligated in an open technique. [5,6,46,41,14] This was modified to a totally endoscopic lateral approach after a learning curve performed by the author: Once the adenoma is dissected, the 10mm endoscope is replaced by a 5mm one. This will facilitate the introduction of a grasper to remove the adenoma through the same trocar. Extraction of small adenomas is usually feasible through the principle 10mm trocar. However, larger ones that cannot be removed through the trocar are usually kept at its tip and removed together while removing the trocar. Routine drainage is not necessary. [41,14] Figure 9.3 shows how the operative field appears with landmarks annotated. This approach has an excellent cure rate (99%), is effective, rapid, bloodless, safe, and has minimum complication rates. With increased experience, it was also possible to operate on associated thyroid pathologies. It was also used in repeat surgery such as a previous contralateral neck surgery or tracheostomy. [43,46,88] However, being a lateral approach, one cannot accomplish a bilateral neck exploration when needed without conversion to open surgery. [41,46]

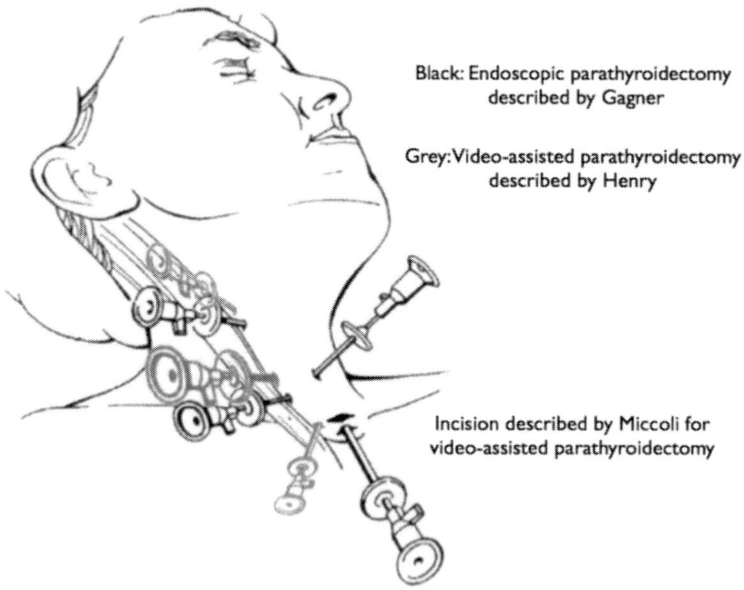

Figure 9.2.

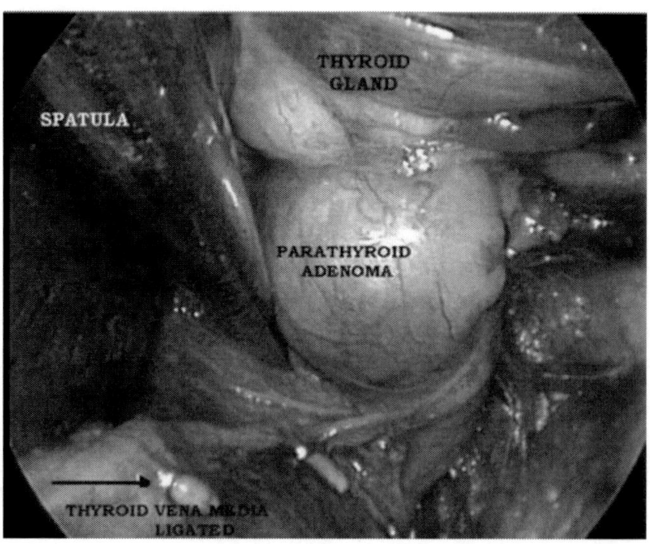

Figure 9.3.

Extracervical Approaches

Minimally invasive surgery of the neck has recently been reported for the treatment of parathyroid diseases. [15] Purely endoscopic parathyroidectomy involves the use of three ports in the neck region, [12,15] and an unwillingness to shift to a purely endoscopic procedure for such a small closed space, the absence of dedicated instruments, and a general concern regarding the effects of constant CO2 insufflation into an extraperitoneal cavity. [15] All of these drawbacks have led other surgeons to attempt a different approach. Some surgeons have devised video-assisted gasless techniques [7,73] or radioguided minimally open surgery. [31] Other surgeons employed incisions made far from the neck region avoiding the problems associated with purely endoscopic techniques. Ikeda and Takami have developed techniques that permit remote access to the neck for either unilateral or bilateral neck exploration. These approaches have the advantage of a larger working space allowing the use of instruments normally used in laparoscopic surgeries. [15,16,17] They have better cosmetic results. Furthermore, the lower CO2 insufflation pressure minimizes its complications. The disadvantages of these techniques include the time required for surgery and the extensive exploration from the anterior chest to the neck, and difficulty in identifying infraclavicular ectopic parathyroid glands. [16]

Anterior Chest Approach

Under general anesthesia, the patient is placed in the supine position with the neck extended. A 5-mm skin incision is made about 3.0 cm below the inferior border of the clavicle, and the lower layer of the platysma is extracted manually. After initiating CO2 insufflation to 4mmHg, a 30° 5-mm endoscope is inserted through the trocar of the side to operate on. Two additional 5-mm trocars are then inserted under endoscopic guidance, one inferior to the sternal notch and the other below the ipsilateral clavicle. The subplatysmal space is developed from the anterior chest.

The thyroid gland is exposed by splitting the sternothyroid muscle, and it is then rotated to reveal the parathyroid glands. The perithyroid fascia is cut carefully to avoid injuring the recurrent laryngeal nerve, so that the parathyroid adenoma protrudes, and the adenoma is then dissected with endoscopic scissors or the Harmonic Scalpel.

The specimen is placed in a finger of a plastic glove and extracted through the 5-mm skin incision. The wound is closed by suturing the adipose tissue with 3-0 absorbable thread, tightly suturing the subcutis with 4-0 absorbable monofilament thread with an atraumatic needle, and then approximating the skin with nonabsorbable thread. [6,15,16] Kitano et al have described a similar gasless technique through the anterior chest wall using a neck region–lifting method. [6,9]

Axillary Approach

Aiming to avoid neck scars, Takami and Ikeda have described a new surgical technique in 2002. [6] Under general anesthesia, the patient is placed in supine position with the neck slightly extended, and the arm on the side of the lesion is raised to fully expose the axilla. A 3 cm incision is then made in the skin of the axilla, and the lower layer of the platysma muscle is dissected to expose the upper layer of the pectoralis major muscle. The incision is extended beneath the skin using a Vein Harvest. A 12-mm and a 5-mm trocar are inserted through the incision, and a purse string suture is made to prevent gas leakage and stop the trocar from slipping out of the wound. Carbon dioxide is insufflated up to a pressure of 4 mmHg. A flexible laparoscope is then inserted through the 12-mm trocar.

A space is created after adequate dissection, and a second 5-mm trocar is inserted near the 3 cm skin incision in the axilla under endoscopic guidance. Endoscopic scissors are used for blunt and sharp dissection to enlarge the subplastymal space. The anterior border of the sternocleidomastoid muscle is dissected from the sternohyoid muscle, and a space is created. The thyroid gland is exposed by splitting the sternothyroid muscle.

The superior or inferior pole of the thyroid gland is then rotated forward to reveal one of the parathyroid glands. The perithyroid fascia is carefully cut so that the parathyroid adenoma protrudes, and the adenoma is dissected using endoscopic scissors or the harmonic scalpel (HS). The other ipsilateral parathyroid gland is also explored. If the parathyroid gland appears normal, a biopsy is performed.

If the gland appears to be enlarged, it is dissected and removed using the endoscopic scissors. The specimen is extracted through the incision in the skin. The wounds are closed with 3-0 absorbable thread sutures after the subcutis had been tightly sutured using a 4-0 absorbable monofilament thread and an atraumatic needle. Tape is used to approximate the skin. [6,17]

Alternative Approaches

The cosmetic implications of neck surgery have motivated surgeons and investigators to develop new approaches to access the neck, skull base, and aerodigestive track using minimally invasive techniques. It's noteworthy to shed some light on the procedures essentially described for thyroidectomy that could be applicable in parathyroid surgery. [18]

The Anterior/Breast Approach

It was first employed by Ohgami et al. in 2000. The subcutaneous space in the breast area and the subplatysmal space in the neck were bluntly dissected through a 15 mm transverse incision at the level of the nipples. CO2 was then insufflated at 6mmHG to create the operative space. Three trocars were then inserted at the breast, and dissection was carried on using an ultrasonically activated scalpel. [18,19]

In 2003, Park et al. used two incisions on each upper circumareolar area. One incision was used for a 12-mm trocar (for endoscopic instruments) and the other for a 15-mm trocar to guide the flexible endoscope. A third incision was made about 3 cm below the clavicle of the tumor side, through which a 5-mm port was inserted. [18,20]

The Axillary-Bilateral Breast Approach (ABBA)

The ABBA was first described in 2003 by Shimazu et al. it has been described as a hybrid procedure combining both axillary and breast approaches. [21] The main reason for this approach is it improves the angulations between the endoscopic instruments relative to the thyroid gland. Under general anesthesia, the patient's neck is slightly extended.

The arm on the tumor side is first abducted, and the legs are parted such that the camera person can stand between the legs. A 2.5 cm incision is made along the upper margin of the areola on the tumor side. After blunt dissection of the subcutaneous tissue of the breast, a subplatysmal working space is created with a balloon dissector.

Following insertion of a 10 mm trocar through the incision, the working space is inflated with CO_2 gas at 4 to 6 mm Hg, and a 10-mm telescope is inserted through the trocar. Two additional 10 mm trocars are inserted through the axillary incision on the tumor side and through the incision at the upper margin of the areola on the opposite side, respectively. The working space is made wide to the level of thyroid cartilage in the upper side and to the medial edge of each SCM in the lateral sides. The strap muscles and SCM are separated gaining access to the target area. [21,22]

In 2008, Bärlehner and Benhidjeb have slightly modified this approach using smaller 5mm trocars and instruments. [22,72] ABBA has the advantage of avoiding the parasternal incision used in the breast approach, which produced hypertrophic scars in a significant number of patients. [18]

The Bilateral Axillo-Breast Approach (BABA)

Choe et al. modified the ABBA in 2007, by developing the BABA. It is also a combined axillary and breast approach, except one more axillary port on the opposite side is inserted. [18,22,23] Under general anesthesia, the patient is placed in supine position with the neck extended using a pillow. Both arms are mildly abducted to provide for insertion of 5 mm ports. Diluted (1:200,000) epinephrine solution is injected into the subcutaneous space in both breasts and the subplatysmal space in the neck to reduce bleeding during dissection. After making two incisions on both upper circumareolar areas, subcutaneous and subplatysmal dissections are performed bluntly with the use of a Rochester clamp and vascular tunneler. The working space is extended to the level of the thyroid cartilage superiorly and to the medial border of each sternocleidomastoid muscle laterally. [22,23] After establishing the required working space, 12 mm ports are inserted. The working space is maintained with CO_2 insufflation at a pressure of 5 to 6 mm Hg. The remaining dissection is completed with the visual guidance of the flexible endoscope. Two 5 mm ports are inserted into each axilla. Strap muscles are split in the middle. Retraction of the thyroid tissue for dissection of its lateral and posterior aspects follows. The procedure is continued in the usual fachion. [18,22,23]

In 2009, Koh et al. published their experience with a unilateral axillo-breast approach without gas insufflation for unilateral benign thyroid lesions. [23b] A skin incision is made in the axilla, 4.5–5.5 cm long and parallel to the skin crease, for insertion of a 10-mm endoscope and instruments. A second skin incision, 1 cm in length, is made along the upper margin of the mammary areola on the tumor side and a 12-mm trocar inserted. [18,23b]

The Postauricular and Axillary Approach (PAA)

In 2009, Lee and colleagues developed a novel endoscopic technique using two axillary and two postauricular ports. He has used it for both thyroid and parathyroid pathologies. [24] This technique avoids excessive dissection around the areolar areas, a major concern for some female patients. [18,22]

Under general endotracheal anesthesia with nasal intubation, the patient is placed in a supine position. [24] The neck is slightly extended and both arms are mildly abducted to provide space for the insertion of the axillary ports. The operator stands on the side of the lesion, the camera is placed on the opposite side, and two assistants are situated at the head of the patient. A 21-gauge spinal needle is used to subcutaneously infiltrate the subplatysmal space of the neck and the subcutaneous space of the axillary and anterior chest area with diluted epinephrine solution (0.1 ml of epinephrine [1:1000] in 200 ml of normal saline). The infiltration provides space for flap dissection and prevents bleeding. A 12-mm axillary incision is made at the lesion side, and the subplatysmal and subcutaneous spaces are dissected bluntly by using a vascular tunneler. The working space is extended superiorly, laterally, and inferiorly to the level of the thyroid cartilage, the medial border of each sternocleidomastoid muscle, and the anterior chest, respectively. [22,24] After establishing the required working space, a 12-mm trocar is inserted and the operative space under the flap is insufflated with low-pressure carbon dioxide gas (5-6 mmHg). Another incision is made on the contralateral axillary region and a 5-mm trocar is inserted. By using 5-mm ultrasonic shears, the rest of the dissection is completed with the visual guidance of a 5-mm flexible videoscope. Bilateral postauricular incisions are then made and two 5-mm trocars are inserted. These are used to aid an incision between the strap muscles and their retraction. The resected specimen is removed through the 12-mm axillary port, contained in a plastic bag. [18,22,24] There have been no cases of facial nerve palsy nor vocal cord paralysis. [18]

Thoracoscopic Approach

Most ectopic parathyroid glands are found in the superior mediastinum within the thymus and can be removed through a cervical incision [25] provided that pre-op localization tests show that the target glands are located 6cm below the clavicular head. [52] On the other hand, in 1% to 2% of patients, the parathyroid migrates deep into the mediastinum or chest being inaccessible through the neck where thoracic approaches as thoracotomy, median sternotomy, or thoracoscopy are required. As expected, those conventional open procedures have a high complication rate and a long recovery time. [25] Other less invasive methods include angiographic ablation, subxiphoid laparoscopy, and mediastinoscopy. [26] In 1994, Prinz et al. performed the first thoracoscopic removal of a mediastinal ectopic hyperfunctioning parathyroid gland. [25] The operation is performed under general anesthesia using a double-lumen endotracheal tube, for single lung ventilation, with the patient placed in the lateral position. [25,26] Three trocar sites are generally used. A camera port is inserted in the seventh intercostals space in the posterior axillary line while light CO_2 insufflation is carried on to decompress the lung. Two additional trocars are then inserted posteriorly and anteriorly. [26] A fourth trocar might be needed for lung retraction. [25] The dissection is carried out using endoscopic instruments. [25] The mediastinal pleura is incised, and the parathyroid is localized on the basis of pre-op localization radiography. The vascular pedicle is interrupted between two metallic clips, and the gland is extracted using an endobag. Any residual CO2 is suctioned prior to removal of the trocars. Chest tubes are not routinely used. [25,26]

Thoracoscopy should not be an exploratory approach; thus, for optimal results, it is recommended to have accurate pre-op localization studies, the best of which is the combination of scintigraphy with CT or MRI. [25]

This procedure is considered safe, provides adequate hemostasis, and provides access to all mediastinal locations of the parathyroids. This procedure also carries minimum post-op complications that are largely limited to minor recurrent effusions, intercostal neuralgia, or correctable hypocalcemia. [25,26] The rate of conversion to an open procedure is low. Post-op hospital stay is short when compared to the thoracotomy or sternotomy. [26]

Da Vinci Robot-Assisted Thoracoscopy: A New Application in Endocrine Surgery

Tele-robotic surgery has inaugurated a new era in minimal invasive surgery with major potential changes concerning concept and performance of surgery itself. This system was primarily developed for cardiac surgery and was the first robotic system to be approved by the Food and Drug Administration for intra-abdominal surgery in the United States in July 2000. [58] Application of the da Vinci system in otolaryngology has been reported in animal models and quite recently in humans. [27,58]

As mentioned earlier, almost all pathologic glands (hyperplasia or adenoma) are located in the neck but 1-2% may be located in the mediastinum and may require a sternotomy or thoracotomy approach for resection. The thoracoscopic approach was proposed in 1994. The DaVinci robotic system allows performance of this thoracoscopic procedure with the benefits of 3-dimensional vision, and improved surgical dexterity and ergonomics. [29]

The da Vinci robot consists of a master console, where the surgeon handles tele-manipulators and optical controls with 3-dimensional vision, and the surgical arm cart, a manipulator unit with two instrument arms and a central arm to guide the two-channel endoscope. The surgeon's movement of the handles is transmitted to the tips of the robotic instruments. The main technologic advantage of this system is that it provides realistic 3-dimensional imaging, motion scaling, and tremor filtration. Thus it allows more precise and accurate endoscopic surgery. The patient is placed in a right lateral decubitus position with contralateral single-lung ventilation. [27,29] A 10-mm port for the robotic endoscope is positioned in the 6th intercostal space in the anterior axillary line, and two 8-mm robotic operating ports are placed in the 4th intercostal space, a handbreadth right and left of the first incision. An accessory port might be placed in the mid-clavicular line through the sixth intercostal space, through which a flexible retractor is inserted to hold the lung away. A second accessory port through the posterior axillary line of the 6th intercostal space might be provided for eventual suction. Resection of the adenoma is performed exclusively by the surgeon at the console. Preparation starts with incision of the parietal pleura covering the aortopulmonary window. The left vagal and recurrent laryngeal nerves are identified. Dissection proceeds beyond the small curvature of the aortic arch towards the trachea. The adenoma is identified adjacent to the trachea between the common trunk of the pulmonary artery and the aorta. Robotic manipulation is performed mainly bluntly with partial use of electrocautery, and care is taken not to rupture the adenoma's capsule. The vascular pedicle is controlled with clips. Minor bleeding from adjacent connective tissue is controlled by compression. Once the adenoma is freed, it is removed with an Endobag system. At the end of the operation, a chest tube is placed.

The resection of a parathyroid from the aortopulmonary window was thus proved to be an ideal case for the robot. The robotic procedure was found to be more accurate and safer than conventional video-assisted thoracoscopic surgery. [27] One of the disadvantages of robotic surgery is its current lack of tactile feedback. However, only about 10% of our sensory system is tactile and 70% to 80% derives from visual input. Thus, a lack of haptic feedback is compensated by the superior image of the three dimensional camera. [28] Another major obstacle for broader application of robotic surgery is, of course, its cost. [28,58] Intraoperative and postoperative complications such as blood loss were comparable with those of conventional thoracoscopic interventions. It has been concluded that robotic surgery combines the advantages of conventional video assisted thoracoscopic surgery (VATS) with the accuracy and safety of an open procedure. [28]

Transoral Approach

Natural orifice transluminal endoscopic surgery (N.O.T.E.S) has been suggested to minimize operative trauma and perioperative morbidity. Additionally, it is aimed towards better cosmetic results. [30,71] Karakas et al have experimented this technique on both living and cadaveric pigs, and human cadavers. [30] Lately, he applied this technique on a living human. [71] The technique described by the author is the following: After a 20-mm paralingual incision of the mucosa on the floor of the mouth, the modified oraloscope is pushed forward by visually controlled blunt dissection of the soft tissue of the neck. Lingual nerve, lingual artery, and lingual branches of the glossopharyngeal nerve or salivary glands are not affected by transection or during careful blunt preparation. The access takes course behind the strap muscles and the hyoid bone following the predetermined embryological way along the thyroglossal duct. Dissecting the tissue within the correct plane the thyroid region is reached without any tissue damage and bleeding. Additional insufflation of carbon dioxide (CO_2) gas to establish a pneumocollum is unnecessary. Maintaining the correct plane behind the hyoid bone and the strap muscles, one is able to reach the dorsolateral space adjacent to the trachea and the posterior aspect of the thyroid gland, considered the key area in thyroid and parathyroid surgery. As an obligatory step before resection of the thyroid and parathyroid glands, a complete dissection of the recurrent laryngeal nerve is performed. Preparation, mobilization, and resection of the glands are performed using conventional 5-mm laparoscopic instruments, whereas blood vessel sealing is achieved with the above-mentioned ultrasonic scissor. Surgery is performed via an entirely transoral sublingual access so that, in contrast to others, an additional medial skin incision below the larynx to insert a small fixation forceps through a trocar is unnecessary. After resection of the parathyroid gland, the sublingual mucosal incision is easily sealed using an absorbable suture. [30] Using this technique, the area of the thyroid region can be reached easily posing less risk to the recurrent laryngeal nerves. Furthermore, it allows for a simple evaluation and localization of all the parathyroid glands without an accessorial skin incision in the neck provided that one is following the naturally predetermined access. [30] Despite the fact that this approach is shifting MIP to a potentially septic surgical intervention, the author did not seem to report any hazardous infectious complication, but this should be further investigated. [30,71] Transoral parathyroidectomy is a promising technique, but it is still in a developmental stage; further evaluations are inevitable to evaluate drawbacks and opportunities. [30]

Minimally Invasive Radioguided Parathyroidectomy (MIRP)

Preoperative localization with MIBI, which has higher sensitivity (90%) than ultrasonography (70–80%), computed tomography (~75–83%), or magnetic resonance imaging (~85%), has revolutionized parathyroidectomy and permitted minimally invasive radioguided surgery (MIRP). [32]

The patient is scanned in the morning. Within 2-3 hours, he is transferred to the operating room. After positioning, an 11mm hand-held gamma probe is used to scan the four quadrants of the neck. [31,32] Incision then guided dissection using the gamma probe determined by the increasing gamma emission to locate the radioactive gland is carried out. The suspected parathyroid is excised. Then, radioactive ratios of the ex-vivo tissue versus background radioactivity are calculated. Parathyroidectomy is considered complete if the excised tissue is morphologically consistent with a parathyroid gland, and contained more than 20% of the background radioactivity. [32,34,35,57]

MIRP has the following potential advantages: (1) localizing the parathyroid adenoma with the in-vivo count; this is equally effective in both positive and negative pre-op sestamibi scan, and it is of special value in ectopic glands and reoperations (previous parathyroidectomies or thyroidectomies where the operative fields is characterized by dense scar tissue), (2) confirming the removal of parathyroid tissue using the ex-vivo count, (3) decreasing the number of frozen sections and qPTH level, (4) decreasing operative and recovery times, and (5) ensuring cure. [34]

Accurate scintigraphy requires dedicated staff. [34] Detailed monitoring of all the potential radiation hazards has shown this procedure to pose no significant risk to operating room personnel, surgeon, or pathologist. The cumulative radiation exposure is relatively insignificant falling within the acceptable yearly exposure as determined by the Nuclear Regulatory Commission. [31]

In conclusion, although the MIRP probe may seem to be a useful tool in parathyroid surgery, its use has not improved the outcome of such surgery. [57] However, it could be beneficial in reoperative neck surgery. [34,70]

Ethanol Ablation

Ultrasound-guided ethanol ablation of culprit parathyroid tissue has been proposed; [69] however, it has a very low cure rate relative to surgical re-exploration. Additionally, recurrent laryngeal nerve (RLN) injury has been reported. It should be reserved for cases in which surgery cannot be safely performed. [3]

Intra-op / quick PTH Level (iPTH, ioPTH, qPTH)

All kinds of focused parathyroidectomies rely on pre-op localization studies and iPTH. Controversies around quick intraoperative PTH assay involve its indications, the criteria for cure, and failures (false decline and false non-decline). [57] The routine use of iPTH improves cure rate of oMIP and VAP when compared to image-guided parathyroidectomy without iPTH (level IV evidence). It also offers a value-adding surgical decision of further neck exploration. Level II evidence suggests that the bilateral exploration during MIVAP permits to avoid both the time and costs of ioPTH with the same effectiveness of endoscopic focused parathyroidectomy with ioPTH monitoring, without prolonging the surgical procedure, but with an increased risk to unnecessarily remove nonpathologic parathyroid glands. In conclusion, there is a grade C recommendation to associate ioPTH monitoring in case of targeted MIVAP and a grade B recommendation to avoid this procedure in case of video-assisted bilateral neck exploration. [41] To obtain a better specificity, it is necessary to extend its sampling period to 20 minutes post excision of the gland. PTH decrease 50% at 20 minutes and/or a significant increase at 20 minutes compared with a 10 minute value are the best predictors of operative failure and multiglandular disease. [41,57]

Negative Pre-op Localization

Negative imaging patients have a higher incidence of multigland disease, lower cure rate, and consume more institutional resources than patients with positive preoperative localization; hence, such patients should be referred to an experienced surgical team. [50] Below, an algorithm for surgical and diagnostic treatment of pHPT has been proposed. (figure 2) [50,66] figure 2 reference 66 (may omit)

MIP: Advantages and Disadvantages

It is not easy to show the meaningful advantages over conventional surgery since the latter has been practiced for a long time with high success rate and minimal mortality and morbidity. The main complications of blood loss, nerve injury, or recurrence are the same as conventional surgery. [38,59] MIP and conventional surgery appear to have similar cure rates. [41] The potential advantage of endoscopic techniques is the greater image provided by magnification and illumination using the endoscope. Whether it is better than a pair of ×2.5 or ×3.5 magnifying loops to identify anatomical structures is difficult to prove. [36,42] Randomized trials have shown that MIP decreases the potential risk of transient post-op hypocalcaemia. [38,41,59] oMIP and MIVAP are more favorable than conventional surgery in terms of operative time. However, in oMIP, surgical exploration is limited and hindered by the length of the skin incision. A prospective randomized trial between MIVAP and oMIP has shown that MIVAP is associated with easier recognition of the recurrent laryngeal nerve. [38] MIP is also superior in terms of cosmetics. [38,41] Knowing that oMIP is performed through a relatively longer incision, especially in obese patients, [38] MIVAP has turned out to be superior to oMIP in terms of scar length and earlier cosmetic results. [41,48] In endoscopic minimally invasive parathyroidectomy (EMIP), one can argue that it requires additional trocars, but these trocars are 2.5–3 mm in section and do not leave any scar in the neck. [36] With MIP, there's a diminution of postoperative pain, earlier recovery, and hence, shorter hospital stay. Operative duration also appears to be shorter except with purely endoscopic techniques. [38,41,59]

Endoscopic and video-assisted surgeries are associated with a steep learning curve. [46] Also, In minimally invasive surgery, which requires creation of the working space for surgical procedures such as neck surgery, the space is likely to be small, making the surgery difficult to perform. [44,46] Furthermore, despite careful selection, multiple glandular disease leading to failed MIP remains a possibility. [40] Conversion is rarely needed for surgical complications such as bleeding or difficult dissection, but more often because of failure to locate the adenoma within a reasonable period of time, difficult dissection, large adenomas taking up most of the working space, fasle-positive imaging studies and inadequate decrease in iPTH level. [43,46,59] Moreover, the risks associated with CO2 insufflation, like hypercarbiarespiratory acidosis, or subcutaneous emphysema, are not completely eliminated. However, insufflation is harmless as long as the procedure is performed under low pressure. [46,59] Potential disadvantages for focused parathyroidectomy, which apply to both open and EMIP approaches, are capsular rupture of adenomas, leading to a condition known as parathyromatosis. [40,41,46,59] Whether endoscopic procedures are less costly than conventional ones is questionable. [53] Finally, it has been found that hyperthyroidism might complicate routine parathyroid operations for HPTH. Knowing that the extent of dissection may play a role, continued efforts to minimize the extent of parathyroid exploration may reduce the potential morbidity of hyperthyroidism after parathyroid exploration. [60]

Recurrent/Persistant PHPT

Persistent HPT is defined as hypercalcemia persisting or recurring within 6 months following surgical exploration, while recurrent HPT is defined as hypercalcemia recurring after 6months of normocalcemia after initial operation. [59] Causes may vary from ectopic locations, parathyromatosis, parathyroid cancer, incomplete resection, supernumerary gland disease. [67,68] No randomized studies have been done to approach patients with recurrent sporadic pHPT. Current recommendation based on case series and expert opinion can be summarized as follows:

1.Concordant functional and anatomic imaging studies should be sought.
2.Whenever possible, a selective image-guided approach is preferred.
3.Judicious use of parathyroid autotransplantation is recommended.
4.Intraoperative PTH assay is recommended to confirm biochemical cure. [59]

Conclusion

Advances in the accuracy of preoperative and peri-operative localizing techniques has lead to a preference for a minimally invasive procedure over bilateral exploration in image localized sporadic primary hyperparathyroidism.

Minimally invasive surgery can be defined as the ability of the surgeon to perform traditional surgical procedures in novel ways to minimize the trauma of the surgical exposure.

MIP may be divided into two groups: mini-open approaches performed under direct vision via a small cervical incision and techniques using the endoscope.

MIP can be done under either general or locoregional anesthesia.

Several other approaches have been also described: from the chest wall, the breast, and the axilla, which has gained its widest acceptance in the Asian community.

The video assisted technique, first described by Miccoli, is a gas-less approach performed through a 1.5cm midline incision located between the cricoid cartilage and the sternal notch. This technique has the advantage of a bilateral exploration from the same incision.

Endoscopic parathyroidectomy by the lateral approach, described by Henry et al., is a total endoscopic approach using gas insufflation and several trocars.

It is best indicated for adenomas that lie deep to the thyroid lobe, usually arising from superior gland adenomas.

All these minimally invasive techniques rely on preoperative localizing studies and may benefit from intra-operative PTH monitoring.

Controversies around quick intraoperative PTH assay involve its indications, the criteria for cure, and failures.

Negative imaging patients should be referred to a specialized surgical team.

MIP and conventional surgery are similar in terms of blood loss, nerve injury, cure rates, and recurrence.

MIP is superior in terms of cosmetics, duration of intervention, post-op stay, and hypocalcaemia as concluded by prospective randomized studies.

References

[1] Naitoh T, Gagner M, Garcia-Ruiz A, Heniford BT. Endoscopic endocrine surgery in the neck. An initial report of endoscopic subtotal parathyroidectomy. *Surg. Endosc.* 1998 Mar;12(3):202-5; discussion 206.

[2] Inabnet WB 3rd, Dakin GF, Haber RS, Rubino F, Diamond EJ, Gagner M. Targeted parathyroidectomy in the era of intraoperative parathormone monitoring. *World J. Surg.* 2002 Aug;26(8):921-5.

[3] Felger EA, Kandil E. Primary hyperparathyroidism. *Otolaryngol. Clin. North Am.* 2010 Apr;43(2):417-32, x.

[4] Lew JI, Solorzano CC. Surgical management of primary hyperparathyroidism: state of the art. *Surg. Clin. North Am.* 2009 Oct;89(5):1205-25.

[5] Osmak-Tizon L, Cougard P. Video-assisted and endoscopic parathyroidectomy and thyroidectomy. Ann Chir. 2006 Jan;131(1):57-61.

[6] Assalia A, Inabnet WB. Endoscopic parathyroidectomy. *Otolaryngol. Clin. North Am.* 2004 Aug;37(4):871-86, xi.

[7] Cougard P, Goudet P, Osmak L, Ferrand L, Letourneau B, Brun JM. Videocervicoscopy in surgery of primary hyperparathyroidism. Preliminary study of 19 patients. *Ann. Chir.* 1998;52(9):885-9.

[8] Cougard P, Goudet P. Video-endoscopic excision of a parathyroid adenoma: surgical technique. *J. Chir.* (Paris). 1999;136(5):264-7.

[9] Usui Y, Sasaki T, Kimura K, Tanaka N, Kotani Y, Saisho S, et al. Gasless endoscopic thyroid and parathyroid surgery using a new retractor. *Surg. Today.* 2001;31(10):939-41.

[10] Cougard P, Goudet P, Bilosi M, Peschaud F. Videoendoscopic approach for parathyroid adenomas: results of a prospective study of 100 patients. *Ann. Chir.* 2001 May;126 (4):314-9.

[11] Yeung GH. Endoscopic surgery of the neck: a new frontier. *Surg. Laparosc. Endosc.* 1998 Jun;8(3):227-32.

[12] Gagner M. Endoscopic subtotal parathyroidectomy in patients with primary hyperparathyroidism. *Br. J. Surg.* 1996 Jun;83(6):875.

[13] Henry JF, Defechereux T, Gramatica L, de Boissezon C. Minimally invasive videoscopic parathyroidectomy by lateral approach. *Langenbecks Arch. Surg.* 1999 Jun;384(3):298-301.

[14] Henry JF, Sebag F, Ippolito G. Endoscopic parathyroidectomy through a lateral approach. *J. Chir.* (Paris). 2008 Sep-Oct;145(5):470-4.

[15] Ikeda Y, Takami H, Niimi M, Kan S, Sasaki Y, Takayama J. Endoscopic total parathyroidectomy by the anterior chest approach for renal hyperparathyroidism. *Surg. Endosc.* 2002 Feb;16(2):320-2.

[16] Ikeda Y, Takami H, Tajima G, Sasaki Y, Takayama J, Kurihara H, et al. Total endoscopic parathyroidectomy. *Biomed. Pharmacother.* 2002;56 Suppl 1:22s-25s.

[17] Ikeda Y, Takami H, Niimi M, Kan S, Sasaki Y, Takayama J. Endoscopic thyroidectomy and parathyroidectomy by the axillary approach. A preliminary report. *Surg. Endosc.* 2002 Jan;16(1):92-5.

[18] Papaspyrou G, Ferlito A, Silver CE, Werner JA, Genden E, Sesterhenn AM. Extracervical approaches to endoscopic thyroid surgery. *Surg. Endosc.* 2010 Sep 16. [Epub ahead of print]

[19] Ohgami M, Ishii S, Arisawa Y, Ohmori T, Noga K, Furukawa T, et al. Scarless endoscopic thyroidectomy: breast approach for better cosmesis. *Surg. Laparosc. Endosc. Percutan. Tech.* 2000 Feb;10(1):1-4.

[20] Park YL, Han WK, Bae WG. 100 cases of endoscopic thyroidectomy: breast approach. *Surg. Laparosc. Endosc. Percutan. Tech.* 2003 Feb;13(1):20-5.

[21] Shimazu K, Shiba E, Tamaki Y, Takiguchi S, Taniguchi E, Ohashi S, et al. Endoscopic thyroid surgery through the axillo-bilateral-breast approach. *Surg. Laparosc. Endosc. Percutan. Tech.* 2003 Jun;13(3):196-201.

[22] Lang BH. Minimally invasive thyroid and parathyroid operations: surgical techniques and pearls. *Adv. Surg.* 2010;44:185-98.

[23] Choe JH, Kim SW, Chung KW, Park KS, Han W, Noh DY, et al. Endoscopic thyroidectomy using a new bilateral axillo-breast approach. *World J. Surg.* 2007 Mar;31(3):601-6.

[24] Koh YW, Kim JW, Lee SW, Choi EC. Endoscopic thyroidectomy via a unilateral axillo-breast approach without gas insufflation for unilateral benign thyroid lesions. *Surg. Endosc.* 2009 Sep;23(9):2053-60. Epub 2008 Jun 5.

[25] Lee KE, Kim HY, Park WS, Choe JH, Kwon MR, Oh SK, et al. Postauricular and axillary approach endoscopic neck surgery: a new technique. *World J. Surg.* 2009 Apr;33(4):767-72.

[26] Alesina PF, Moka D, Mahlstedt J, Walz MK. Thoracoscopic removal of mediastinal hyperfunctioning parathyroid glands: personal experience and review of the literature. *World J. Surg.* 2008 Feb;32(2):224-31.

[27] Chae AW, Perricone A, Brumund KT, Bouvet M. Outpatient video-assisted thoracoscopic surgery (VATS) for ectopic mediastinal parathyroid adenoma: a case report and review of the literature. *J. Laparoendosc. Adv. Surg. Tech. A.* 2008 Jun;18(3):383-90.

[28] Bodner J, Profanter C, Prommegger R, Greiner A, Margreiter R, Schmid T. Mediastinal parathyroidectomy with the da Vinci robot: presentation of a new technique. *J. Thorac. Cardiovasc. Surg.* 2004 Jun;127(6):1831-2.

[29] Bodner J, Wykypiel H, Greiner A, Kirchmayr W, Freund MC, Margreiter R, et al. Early experience with robot-assisted surgery for mediastinal masses. *Ann. Thorac. Surg.* 2004 Jul;78(1):259-65; discussion 265-6.

[30] Brunaud L, Ayav A, Bresler L, Schjött B. Da Vinci robot-assisted thoracoscopy for primary hyperparathyroidism: a new application in endocrine surgery. *J. Chir.* (Paris). 2008 Mar-Apr;145(2):165-7.

[31] Karakas E, Steinfeldt T, Gockel A, Westermann R, Kiefer A, Bartsch DK. Transoral thyroid and parathyroid surgery. *Surg. Endosc.* 2010 Jun;24(6):1261-7.

[32] Norman J, Chheda H. Minimally invasive parathyroidectomy facilitated by intraoperative nuclear mapping. *Surgery.* 1997 Dec;122(6):998-1003; discussion 1003-4.

[33] McGreal G, Winter DC, Sookhai S, Evoy D, Ryan M, O'Sullivan GC, et al. Minimally invasive, radioguided surgery for primary hyperparathyroidism. *Ann. Surg. Oncol.* 2001 Dec;8(10):856-60.

[34] Dackiw AP, Sussman JJ, Fritsche HA Jr, Delpassand ES, Stanford P, Hoff A, et al. Relative contributions of technetium Tc 99m sestamibi scintigraphy, intraoperative gamma probe detection, and the rapid parathyroid hormone assay to the surgical management of hyperparathyroidism. *Arch. Surg.* 2000 May;135(5):550-5; discussion 555-7.

[35] Jaskowiak NT, Sugg SL, Helke J, Koka MR, Kaplan EL. Pitfalls of intraoperative quick parathyroid hormone monitoring and gamma probe localization in surgery for primary hyperparathyroidism. *Arch. Surg.* 2002 Jun;137(6):659-68; discussion 668-9.

[36] Chen H, Sippel RS, Schaefer S. The effectiveness of radioguided parathyroidectomy in patients with negative technetium tc 99m-sestamibi scans. *Arch. Surg.* 2009 Jul;144(7):643-8.

[37] Henry JF. Minimally invasive thyroid and parathyroid surgery is not a question of length of the incision. *Langenbecks Arch. Surg.* 2008 Sep;393(5):621-6.

[38] Pitale A, Andrabi SI, Dolan SJ, Russell CF. Minimally invasive parathyroid exploration for solitary adenoma. Initial experience with an open, 'short incision' approach. *Ulster. Med. J.* 2008 May;77(2):115-8.

[39] Barczyński M, Cichoń S, Konturek A, Cichoń W. Minimally invasive video-assisted parathyroidectomy versus open minimally invasive parathyroidectomy for a solitary parathyroid adenoma: a prospective, randomized, blinded trial. *World J. Surg.* 2006 May;30(5):721-31.

[40] Udelsman R, Donovan PI, Sokoll LJ. One hundred consecutive minimally invasive parathyroid explorations. *Ann. Surg.* 2000 Sep;232(3):331-9.

[41] Sackett WR, Barraclough B, Reeve TS, Delbridge LW. Worldwide trends in the surgical treatment of primary hyperparathyroidism in the era of minimally invasive parathyroidectomy.*Arch. Surg.* 2002 Sep;137(9):1055-9.

[42] Lombardi CP, Raffaelli M, Traini E, De Crea C, Corsello SM, Bellantone R. Video-assisted minimally invasive parathyroidectomy: benefits and long-term results. *World J. Surg.* 2009 Nov;33(11):2266-81.

[43] Henry JF, Sebag F, Cherenko M, Ippolito G, Taieb D, Vaillant J. Endoscopic parathyroidectomy: why and when? *World J. Surg*. 2008 Nov;32(11):2509-15.

[44] Berti P, Materazzi G, Picone A, Miccoli P. Limits and drawbacks of video-assisted parathyroidectomy. *Br. J. Surg*. 2003 Jun;90(6):743-7.

[45] Rulli F, Galatà G, Pompeo E, Farinon AM. A camera handler for Miccoli's minimally invasive video-assisted thyroidectomy and paratiroidectomy procedures. *Surg. Endosc*. 2007 Jun;21(6):1017-9.

[46] Miccoli P, Berti P, Materazzi G, Ambrosini CE, Fregoli L, Donatini G. Endoscopic bilateral neck exploration versus quick intraoperative parathormone assay (qPTHa) during endoscopic parathyroidectomy: A prospective randomized trial. *Surg. Endosc*. 2008 Feb;22(2):398-400.

[47] Henry JF, Sebag F, Tamagnini P, Forman C, Silaghi H. Endoscopic parathyroid surgery: results of 365 consecutive procedures. *World J. Surg*. 2004 Dec;28(12):1219-23.

[48] Miccoli P, Berti P, Materazzi G, Donatini G. Minimally invasive video assisted parathyroidectomy (MIVAP). *Eur. J. Surg. Oncol*. 2003 Mar;29(2):188-90.

[49] Casserly P, Timon C. Minimally invasive video-assisted parathyroidectomy. *Laryngoscope*. 2009 May;119(5):880-2.

[50] Barbaros U, Erbil Y, Yildirim A, Saricam G, Yazici H, Ozarmağan S. Minimally invasive video-assisted subtotal parathyroidectomy with thymectomy for secondary hyperparathyroidism. *Langenbecks Arch. Surg*. 2009 May;394(3):451-5.

[51] Harari A, Allendorf J, Shifrin A, DiGorgi M, Inabnet WB. Negative preoperative localization leads to greater resource use in the era of minimally invasive parathyroidectomy. *Am. J. Surg*. 2009 Jun;197(6):769-73.

[52] Miccoli P, Berti P, Materazzi G, Massi M, Picone A, Minuto MN. Results of video-assisted parathyroidectomy: single institution's six-year experience. *World J. Surg*. 2004 Dec;28(12):1216-8.

[53] Callender GG, Grubbs EG, Vu T, Hofstetter WL, Fleming JB, Woodburn KL, et al. The fallen one: the inferior parathyroid gland that descends into the mediastinum. *J. Am. Coll. Surg*. 2009 May;208(5):887-93; discussion 893-5.

[54] Miccoli P, Bendinelli C, Berti P, Vignali E, Pinchera A, Marcocci C. Video-assisted versus conventional parathyroidectomy in primary hyperparathyroidism: a prospective randomized study. *Surgery*. 1999 Dec;126(6):1117-21; discussion 1121-2.

[55] Lorenz K, Phuong NT, Dralle H. Diversification of minimally invasive parathyroidectomy for primary hyperparathyroidism: minimally invasive video-assisted parathyroidectomy and minimally invasive open videoscopically magnified parathyroidectomy with local anesthesia. *World J. Surg*. 2002 Aug;26(8):1066-70.

[56] Kitagawa W, Shimizu K, Kumita S, Akasu H, Kumazaki T, Tanaka S. Radio-guided parathyroidectomy for primary hyperparathyroidism combined with video-assisted surgery using the solid-state, multi-crystal gamma camera. *J. Surg. Oncol*. 2002 Jul;80(3):173-5.

[57] De Pasquale L, Bianchi P, Barabino M, Bestetti A, Bastagli A. Radio-guided video-assisted parathyroidectomy: a preliminary report. *Surg. Endosc*. 2001 Dec;15(12):1456-8.

[58] Sitges-Serra A, Rosa P, Valero M, Membrilla E, Sancho JJ. Surgery for sporadic primary hyperparathyroidism: controversies and evidence-based approach. *Langenbecks Arch. Surg.* 2008 May;393(3):239-44.

[59] Braumann C, Jacobi CA, Menenakos C, Ismail M, Rueckert JC, Mueller JM. Robotic-assisted laparoscopic and thoracoscopic surgery with the da Vinci system: a 4-year experience in a single institution. *Surg. Laparosc. Endosc. Percutan. Tech.* 2008 Jun;18(3):260-6.

[60] Mihai R, Barczynski M, Iacobone M, Sitges-Serra A. Surgical strategy for sporadic primary hyperparathyroidism an evidence-based approach to surgical strategy, patient selection, surgical access, and reoperations. *Langenbecks Arch. Surg.* 2009 Sep;394(5):785-98.

[61] Stang MT, Yim JH, Challinor SM, Bahl S, Carty SE. Hyperthyroidism after parathyroid exploration. *Surgery.* 2005 Dec;138(6):1058-64; discussion 1064-5.

[62] Bergenfelz A, Lindblom P, Tibblin S, Westerdahl J. Unilateral versus bilateral neck exploration for primary hyperparathyroidism: a prospective randomized controlled trial. *Ann. Surg.* 2002 Nov;236(5):543-51.

[63] Russell CF, Dolan SJ, Laird JD. Randomized clinical trial comparing scan-directed unilateral versus bilateral cervical exploration for primary hyperparathyroidism due to solitary adenoma. *Br. J. Surg.* 2006 Apr;93(4):418-21.

[64] Palazzo FF, Delbridge LW. Minimal-access/minimally invasive parathyroidectomy for primary hyperparathyroidism. *Surg. Clin. North Am.* 2004 Jun;84(3):717-34.

[65] Barczynski M, Konturek A, Cichon S, Hubalewska-Dydejczyk A, Golkowski F, Huszno B. Intraoperative parathyroid hormone assay improves outcomes of minimally invasive parathyroidectomy mainly in patients with a presumed solitary parathyroid adenoma and missing concordance of preoperative imaging. *Clin. Endocrinol.* (Oxf). 2007 Jun;66(6):878-85.

[66] Sun Y, Cai H, Bai J, Zhao H, Miao Y. Endoscopic total parathyroidectomy and partial parathyroid tissue autotransplantation for patients with secondary hyperparathyroidism: a new surgical approach. *World J. Surg.* 2009 Aug;33(8):1674-9.

[67] Kirkby-Bott J , El-Khatib Z. Recent Advances in Parathyroid Surgery. In: Johnson CD, Taylor I, editors. *Recent Advances of Surgery.* 33rd ed. 2010, page 29-42.

[68] Mariette C, Pellissier L, Combemale F, Quievreux JL, Carnaille B, Proye C. Reoperation for persistent or recurrent primary hyperparathyroidism. *Langenbecks Arch. Surg.* 1998 Apr;383(2):174-9.

[69] Shen W, Düren M, Morita E, Higgins C, Duh QY, Siperstein AE et al. Reoperation for persistent or recurrent primary hyperparathyroidism. *Arch. Surg.* 1996 Aug;131(8):861-7; discussion 867-9.

[70] Harman CR, Grant CS, Hay ID, Hurley DL, van Heerden JA, Thompson GB, et al. Indications, technique, and efficacy of alcohol injection of enlarged parathyroid glands in patients with primary hyperparathyroidism. *Surgery.* 1998 Dec;124(6):1011-9; discussion 1019-20.

[71] Lokey J, Mondragon-Sanchez A, Salazar Navarro F, Pattou F, Carnaille B, Huglo D, et al. Radioguided surgery for primary hyperparathyroidism. Experience in 75 cases. *Ann. Chir.* 2001 Jul;126(6):535-40.

[72] Karakas E, Steinfeldt T, Gockel A, Sesterhenn A, Bartsch DK. Transoral partial parathyroidectomy. *Chirurg.* 2010 Nov;81(11):1020-5.

[73] Bärlehner E, Benhidjeb T. Cervical scarless endoscopic thyroidectomy: Axillo-bilateral-breast approach (ABBA). *Surg. Endosc.* 2008 Jan;22(1):154-7. Epub 2007 Apr 13.

[74] Miccoli P, Bendinelli C, Vignali E, Mazzeo S, Cecchini GM, Pinchera A, et al. Endoscopic parathyroidectomy: report of an initial experience. *Surgery.* 1998 Dec;124(6):1077-9; discussion 1079-80.

[75] Mandl F. Therapeutischer Versuch bei Ostitis fibrosa generalisata mittels Exstirpation eine Epithelkör- perchens. *Wien Klin. Wochenschr.* 1925; 38:1343–1344

[76] Roth SI, Wang CA, Potts JT Jr. The team approach to primary hyperparathyroidism. *Hum. Pathol.* 1975 Nov;6(6):645-8.

[77] Tibblin S, Bondeson AG, Ljungberg O. Unilateral parathyroidectomy in hyperparathyroidism due to single adenoma. *Ann. Surg.* 1982 Mar;195(3):245-52.

[78] Smith JC, Evans LM, Cockcroft JR, Davies JS. Impaired vascular reactivity in primary hyperparathyroidism may contribute to cardiovascular risk. *Clin. Endocrinol.* (Oxf). 2001 Aug;55(2):279-80.

[79] Kautzky-Willer A, Pacini G, Niederle B, Schernthaner G, Prager R. Insulin secretion, insulin sensitivity and hepatic insulin extraction in primary hyperparathyroidism before and after surgery. *Clin. Endocrinol.* (Oxf). 1992 Aug;37(2):147-55.

[80] Cheung PS, Thompson NW, Brothers TE, Vinik AI. Effect of hyperparathyroidism on the control of diabetes mellitus. *Surgery.* 1986 Dec;100(6):1039-47.

[81] Prager R, Schernthaner G, Niederle B, Roka R. Evaluation of glucose tolerance, insulin secretion, and insulin action in patients with primary hyperparathyroidism before and after surgery. Calcif Tissue Int. 1990 Jan;46(1):1-4.

[82] Talpos GB, Bone HG 3rd, Kleerekoper M, Phillips ER, Alam M, Honasoge M, et al. Randomized trial of parathyroidectomy in mild asymptomatic primary hyperparathyroidism: patient description and effects on the SF-36 health survey. *Surgery.* 2000 Dec;128(6):1013-20;discussion 1020-1.

[83] Brunaud L, Zarnegar R, Wada N, Ituarte P, Clark OH, Duh QY. Incision length for standard thyroidectomy and parathyroidectomy: when is it minimally invasive? *Arch. Surg.* 2003 Oct;138(10):1140-3.

[84] Hunter JG. Minimally invasive surgery: the next frontier. *World J. Surg.* 1999 Apr;23(4):422-4.

[85] Carling T, Donovan P, Rinder C, Udelsman R. Minimally invasive parathyroidectomy using cervical block: reasons for conversion to general anesthesia. *Arch. Surg.* 2006 Apr;141(4):401-4; discussion 404.

[86] Donati F, Plaud B. Tracheal intubation: optimal conditions, vocal cord damage, and allergy. *Can. J. Anaesth.* 2008 Oct;55(10):663-9.

[87] Miccoli P, Bendinelli C, Conte M et al (1998) Endoscopic parathyroidectomy by a gasless approach. *J. Laparoendosc. Adv. Surg. Tech. A* 8:189–194.

[88] Lorenz K, Miccoli P, Monchik JM, Düren M, Dralle H. Minimally invasive video-assisted parathyroidectomy: multiinstitutional study. *World J. Surg.* 2001 Jun;25(6):704-7.

[89] Henry JF, Iacobone M, Mirallie E, Deveze A, Pili S. Indications and results of video-assisted parathyroidectomy by a lateral approach in patients with primary hyperparathyroidism. *Surgery.* 2001 Dec;130(6):999-1004.

In: Parathyroid: Anatomy, Functions and Disorders
Editor: James Kirkby-Bott
ISBN: 978-1-62100-765-4

Chapter X

Secondary and Tertiary HPT

Gianluca Donatini and Bruno Carnaille
Service de Chirurgie Endocrinienne et metabolique, CHU Lille, France

Abstract

Secondary and tertiary HPT are consequences of renal failure. 1,25 Vitamin D deficiency is associated with parathyroid hyperplasia and is a consequence of renal failure as conversion from 25 OH cholecalciferol to 1,25 dihydroxycholecalciferol, the active form of vitamin D, occurs in the renal parenchyma.

Secondary and Tertiary HPT refer to nodular multigland hyperplasia with excessive over secretion of PTH. This causes ectopic calcification and bone demineralization and hastens declining renal function due to nephrocalcinosis, causing concern for subsequent graft function in transplanted patients who have excessive PTH production at the time of surgery and or develop tertiary HPT post transplantation. Medical treatment with calcimimetics has not been as successful as first hoped and surgery remains the cornerstone treatment of secondary HPT.

There is debate as to the best surgical strategy sub-total parathyroidectomy and total parathyroidectomy +/- auto transplantation and cryopreservation of parathyroid tissue all have their own benefits and drawbacks.

Introduction

Chronic Renal Failure (CRF) is a condition characterized by a glomerular filtration rate (GFR) $<60 mL/min/1.73 m^2$ for ≥ 3 months with demonstrable kidney damage (pathological damage, abnormalities in blood/urine or in imaging studies)[1]. Patients affected by CRF suffer a loss of the homeostatic control of calcium, phosphorus and reduced production of vitamin 1,25 $(OH)_2D_3$ (Calcitriol). The disruption of such balance leads to an increased secretion of parathyroid hormone (PTH), causing hyperplastic growth of the parathyroid glands, and the development of secondary hyperparathyroidism (sHPT) [2]. Given the etiology sHPT is also commonly reported as renal hyperparathyroidism[1,2]. Even though

CRF is the most important factor, other conditions may generate parathyroid hyperplasia: hypermagnesiuria, osteomalacia, malnutrition, idiopathic hypercalciuria, familial hypocalciuric hypercalcemia (FHH), vitamin D deficiency, chronic lithium therapy[3]. Tertiary Hyperparathyroidism (tHPT) refers, instead, to a condition that develops in patients in whom a kidney transplant has been made, but the normalization of renal function fails to control PTH production, which has become autonomous and thus unresponsive to normal or high calcium serum levels. This condition affects as many as 30% of transplanted patients[4,5]. The metabolic dishomeostasis of tHPT may generate significant complications to the transplanted patients ranging from a worsening of a pre-existent skeletal disease up to early loss of the graft, usually through an accelerated nephrocalcinosis[4-6].

Pathogenesis of Secondary Hyperparathyroidism

Many factors explain the development of sHPT: decreased production of 1,25 $(OH)_2D_3$ (Calcitriol), hypocalcemia, phosphate retention, bone resistance to PTH action and PTH set-point change[1,2,7].

1) *Calcitriol crash.* Calcitriol is exclusively produced within the kidney[7]. Its production is stimulated by PTH, which increases activity of renal 1α-hydroxylase needed to convert the 25 (OH) D_3 into the active form, 1,25 dihydroxy D_3. Calcitriol exerts its activity on the bone, intestine, kidney and also the parathyroid glands. On the bone it mobilizes calcium enhancing both the osteoclastic and the osteoblastic activities[8]. In the gut it promotes intestinal absorption of calcium, via a higher expression of the calbindin (calcium binding protein), while in the kidney it stimulates phosphate excretion. Calcitriol also inhibits PTH secretion by increasing the sensitivity of parathyroid cells to calcium levels, reducing cell proliferation and PTH gene expression[7-9]. In CRF Calcitriol levels are lowered as there is little 1α-hydroxylase activity: bone calcium mobilization is impaired, renal reabsorption of phosphate is enhanced, calcium absorption is decreased and the suppressive action of calcitriol on PTH production is lost[10,11].
2) Hypocalcemia. Although sHPT develops early in patients affected by CRF, hypocalcemia may not be present in initial phases[7]. It is the result of combined low Calcitriol levels, hyperphosphatemia and bone resistance to PTH[2,4,7]. In CRF, in fact, serum calcium balance is maintained by a gradually increased PTH secretion, which acts by enhancing bone reabsorption, calcium intestinal absorption and stimulating the renal synthesis of calcitriol[2,7]. Calcium is a key factor in the progression of sHPT. Binding the calcium sensing receptor on parathyroid cells (CaRs) calcium inhibits PTH mRNA synthesis; conversely a prolonged hypocalcemia stimulates PTH secretion leading to parathyroid hyperplasia[12,13].
3) Hyperphosphatemia. Phosphorus acts directly on parathyroid cells to increase synthesis and release of PTH via a post-transcriptional mechanism[14-16]. Dietary phosphate intake in patients with CRF adds to the effect of a reduced kidney excretion[2]. Hyperphosphatemia inhibits Calcitriol production and impairs PTH action on bone, thus contributing to the hypocalcaemic state of patients with CRF and leading to the development of sHPT[14,15].

4) PTH increase. PTH induces bone remodeling, liberating calcium via the activity of osteoclasts, and probably working in concert with calcitriol[12]. Nevertheless in patients with CRF, even an intravenous injection of PTH does not increase significantly serum calcium concentration. This flat response to hormonal stimulation may find answer in the fact that those patients usually have low Calcitriol levels (which prevents osteoclasts activation), hyperphosphatemia and down-regulation of the PTH bone receptor[16,17]. This increasing bone resistance to PTH leads to a perpetuous circle of increased need of PTH to maintain adequate calcium levels, resulting in parathyroid hyperplasia and progressive bone demineralization[2,7].
5) Parathyroid hormone set point. It is defined as the serum calcium concentration capable of determining a decrease of PTH level by 50% [18]. The set point progressively shifts, while CRF is developing, recognizing in the early stages a relative insensitivity to suppression in parathyroid cell activity by calcium serum level, while in advanced stages it relates more with the chronic bone resistance and low levels of calcitriol[19,20]. The latter affects the expression of the calcium sensing receptor on the membrane of parathyroid cells, which is reduced, increasing then the resistance to calcium concentration. The expression of Calcitriol receptors on the membrane surface is also diminished, leading to an increased resistance to Calcitriol. Therefore excessive PTH is secreted at any given serum calcium concentration[20].

Clinical Manifestation of sHPT

The impaired calcium homeostasis in patients with sHPT leads to a significant morbidity and mortality. Clinical manifestations include: musculo-skeletal disease, extra skeletal calcification, pruritus, anemia, hypertension and calciphylaxis.

Renal osteodystrophy is a common and potentially debilitating complication of secondary HPT Bone disease begins early in CRF and musculoskeletal pathologies importantly reduced patient's quality of life. In adults, bone pain mainly in the lower back, hips and legs is a frequent symptom, while fractures may affect long bones, vertebrae and ribs, leading to deformities, represented mainly by kyphosis and lumbar scoliosis. In children, growth retardation is commonly seen; skeletal deformities are frequent due to the intense bone remodeling[21]. Patients with CRF may exhibit a wide spectrum of bone disorders. Bone disease may be classified based on its turnover. The high turnover disease affects those patients in whom high levels of PTH are present. Osteoblastic and osteoclastic activities are both enhanced leading to an accelerated bone reabsorption and formation of woven bone that replaces normal lamellar bone. In a long-standing condition the collagen deposition creates fibrosis and cysts replacing the bone marrow, creating a fragile structure prone to fractures (*Osteitis fibrosa cystica*). It's reported in literature in up to 75% of dialyzed patients[2,22-24]. The lower turnover disease is instead represented by relatively low levels of PTH, a paucity of bone cells and a massive decrease of the active bone remodeling sites. This condition is present in up to 50% of haemodialized patients and it's sustained mainly by an over suppression of PTH by high-calcium dialysates, phosphate binders, Calcitriol and its analogs[2, 24,25]. This group of patients tends to have a hypercalcaemic state with aged bone due to a slow to absent bone remodeling and is at higher risk for fractures[26,27]. In low turnover bone disease two subgroups may be distinct: in the first one a decreased bone formation is coupled with a reduced mineralization (*adynamic bone syndrome*), whereas in the second subgroup the impaired mineralization precedes the decreased collagen deposition (*osteomalacia*). Most uraemic patients, present with a mixed form[27]. Radiological evaluation by means of plan X-ray usually shows subperiostal resorption in the distal phalanx, skull, clavicle, ribs and femur as well as ill-defined bands of increased bone density adjacent to the vertebral endplate[22-27].

Extra skeletal calcifications usually develop in patients with a high calcium / phosphorus product and may localize in three different settings: visceral, vascular and periarticular. *Visceral calcifications* may affect the lung (causing restrictive disease), the heart (leading to left ventricular hypertrophy and heart dysfunction), mitral valve, skeletal muscle, breast, stomach, and the eye[28-32]. Within this group of patients a particular clinical feature is represented by *red eye*[33,34]. It's characterized by a diffuse waxy red episcleral and conjunctival hyperaemia extending beyond the palpebral angle with little or no exudates[33].

Conjuntival thickening with red eye (81.3%) is a common finding, being present in up to 80% of dialyzed patients[34]. It's related to a disturbance of the calcium metabolism: serum calcium and phosphate levels are positively correlated with the degree of conjunctival calcification[33,34].

A correct control of serum calcium concentration significantly improves this condition, with disappearance of red eye and decreased conjuntival thickness[33,34]. Peyronies disease due to penile calcifications causing sexual dysfunction has also been observed[35].

Vascular calcifications localize in both large and small vessels and the prevalence is up to 20% in patients with end stage CRF[36]. *Periarticular calcifications* usually affect small-joints causing periarthritis and peri-articular effusions. These alterations are shown by X-ray examination. Parathyroidectomy does not improve vascular calcifications whilst it diminishes extra-vascular calcifications.

Arterial hypertension, frequently, is cause and effect of CRF. It has been observed that intracellular calcium levels are altered in salt dependent types of hypertension. Among patients with CRF those with overt sHPT have the highest levels of both arterial blood pressure and intracellular calcium concentration[37,38]. Parathyroidectomy positively affects hypertension[39].

Another extremely frequent condition in CRF is *pruritus*, reported up to 85% of haemodialized patients. Its etiology seems to correlate with levels of calcium, phosphate, mag-nesium and their ionic products rather than with a direct action of PTH. Nevertheless after parathyroidectomy patients exhibit a dramatic improvement of pruritus[40,41].

Normocromic, normocytic *anemia* is common in CRF, due to the lack of secretion of erythropoietin, iron deficiency, aluminium toxicity and recurrent infection. PTH hyper-secretion may by itself complicate the anemia by reducing erythropoietin synthesis, shortening red blood cell life span and producing bone marrow fibrosis[42].

Calciphylaxis is a severe and potentially lethal complication of sHPT. This uncommon syndrome is characterized by diffuse calcification of both soft and small arterioles leading to tissue necrosis. Clinically the patients appear with painful lilaceous, mottled lesions that progress deeply causing areas of non-healing wounds and gangrene. This lesion may become complicated by wound infections and sepsis.

The prognosis is poor with mortality as high as 50%. Usually these patients present with a high Calcium X Phosphorus product, whilst PTH may not be too elevated. A mathematical model has been prepared to identify patients at risk of calciphylaxis[4,43]. When such symptoms are present, patients might be treated with phosphate binders and timely total parathyroidectomy[4,44,45].

Management of Renal Hyperparathyroidism and Its Role in Relation to Renal Transplant

The main treatment for sHPT is medical[46]. It should be started as early as possible in CRF to prevent progression of sHPT and thus its complications. In early stages, oral calcium and vitamin D supplementation is sufficient to correct calcium/phosphorus homeostasis thus reducing PTH levels[2,4,46-48]. Later, calcimimetics, phosphate binders (such as Sevelamer) and vitamin D analogues may be used to achieve a better control of sHPT[46-50]. In end-stage CRF patients a careful balance of aluminium and other binding agents in the dialyzing medium may reduce the incidence of sHPT[46,47].

Medical treatments goal is to achieve a good control of sHPT and, whenever possible, to bridge the patient to a transplant, which is, the optimal and definitive treatment for sHPT[2,4,46,47].

Even though the recent introduction of calcimimetics into medical therapy, has produced great results in controlling PTH secretion, up to 5% of dialysis patients require surgical treatment per annum[2,4,46]. As stated by the K/DOQI guidelines[46], surgical indications are represented by:

1) Failure of medical therapy (PTH levels 800 pg/mL, hypercalcemia, hyperphosphatemia or complications of sHPT (pruritus, bone fractures, ectopic calcifications).
2) Calciphylaxis with PTH levels 500 pg/ml

Tertiary HPT (tHPT), as previously stated, may have a prevalence of up to 30% of transplanted patients[4-6,51]. Tertiary hyperparathyroidism is commonly due to parathyroid hyperplasia involving 1 or more glands. Some investigators have reported that 2.6% to 32% of tHPT may be due to a single adenoma or double adenomas[51,52]. Generally, operative intervention is recommended in patients with tHPT with, as follows: asymptomatic disease with total calcium level greater than 12.0 mg/dL (3.0 mmol/L) for more than 1 year, acute hypercalcemia or symptomatic hypercalcemia[4,5,51-53]. Some authors consider an early cut-off (more than 3 month of hypercalcemia after the graft), given the fact that if tHPT does develop, earlier surgery will improve the overall outcome, including a preserved function of the grafted kidney [52]. Indeed patients with persistently elevated PTH levels after transplantation are at greater risk for acute tubular necrosis[53] and nephrocalcinosis causing chronic loss of graft function. Additionally parathyroidectomy has been proposed if parathyroid glands weight exceeds 500 mg on ultrasound examinations[4,6]. Nevertheless evidence-based guidelines for the surgical treatment of tHPT have not been established [4,6,52,54].

Preoperative Localization

Pre-operative imaging is not routinely required at the first operation[55]. Patients on dialysis with sHPT always have parathyroid hyperplasia, those not on dialysis usually don't. 99mTc MIBI-scintigraphy scan has a low accuracy rate not exceeding a sensitivity of 40% prior to the first operation[4,55]. Conversely, when a re-operation is performed, MIBI scan may be helpful to find the source of persistence/recurrence if a sub-total parathyroidectomy was the first operation[55-57]. Neck ultrasound examination (US) has also poor accuracy in sHPT and tHPT. Many patients have associated thyroid nodules that decrease specificity of the US exam for parathyroid identification and up to 38% of patient have an ectopic hyperplastic gland[4]; US doesn't scan the anterior mediastinum where an ectopic hyperplastic parathyroid is usually found[54,55]. CT and MRI scan have be used in these cases, although the outcome is unreported, but they help identify ectopic positions such as mediastinal parathyroids[54,55].

Surgical Strategy

The surgical goal in sHPT and tHPT is to reduce the production of PTH. Depending on different experiences and patients' clinical data, there are three possible surgical techniques for parathyroidectomy: sub-total parathyroidectomy (sPTX) [6,53-61], total parathyroidectomy with auto transplantation (PTX + AT)[58-60,62-64] or total parathyroidectomy without auto transplantation (PTX) [60,63-68]. Removed parathyroid tissue, may also be cryopreserved, thus allowing (late) autotransplantation[69,70]. Bilateral cervical thymectomy is always performed both in sPTX and PTX[53-68]. Finding a "hot spot" within the mediastinum will not alter the initial surgical strategy. No indication exists to perform a sternotomy or thoracic approach at the first operation. Moreover patients affected by sHPT have bone disease and that will hamper healing[55,57,63,71-73].

Surgical Technique: Bilateral Neck Exploration

A conventional cervicotomy (Kocher incision's) is made and a thorough bilateral cervical neck exploration is performed to identify at least four parathyroid glands. The procedure must be conducted with meticulous haemostasis, thus allowing easy recognition of the parathyroid glands. Careful dissection is mandatory, to avoid parathyroid capsule rupture and therefore seeding of parathyroid cells which may lead to recurrence (parathyromatosis)[73,74]. Bilateral transcervical thymectomy is performed, to avoid persistence/recurrence by an ectopic supernumerary thymic gland[4,58-60,73]. At this point in time the surgeon has the chance to tailor the surgical procedure to the patient, weighing the pros and cons of the three different approaches.

Sub-Total Parathyroidectomy (sPTX)

Once all the parathyroid glands had been recognized, the least hyperplastic and least nodular gland is excised leaving in situ a fragment of about 50 to 100 mg (twice the size of a normal parathyroid). After this step the three larger glands have to be removed[54,58,59,61]. We strongly support confirming identification of all 4 glands in order to assess correct vascularization of the parathyroid remnant before all other glands are excised. A vascular clip and non absorbable suture are left on the remnant to make an eventual reoperation for recurrent disease easier. It is favorable to choose a gland far from the recurrent laryngeal nerve (usually an inferior gland), to reduce possible injury in case of re-operation, however this decision has be balanced with leaving a relatively normal gland fragment as in those not due to have renal transplantation this can extend the period of time till recurrence due to hyperplastic change in the remnant occurs.

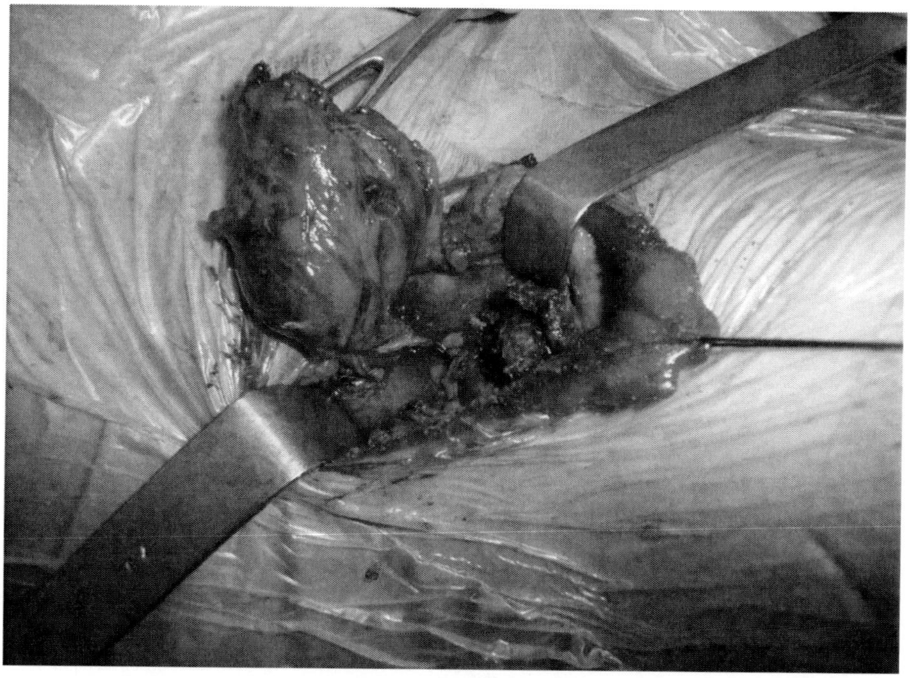

Figure 10.1. Large slightly nodular parathyroid gland in a patient undergoing sub-total parathyroidectomy for renal HPT.

A part of the resected glands may by cryopreserved for delayed transplantation in case of post-operative hypoparathyroidism[69,70]. This operation usually achieves a great reduction of PTH levels coupled with a low rate of post-operative hypocalcemia; it allows early renal grafting. On the other hand recurrence is frequent if CRF is not corrected[4,67]. Figures 10.1 and 10.2 show a nodular hyperplastic parathyroid due to renal HPT and an outline of a sub-total parathyroidectomy.

Total Parathyroidectomy with Auto Transplantation (PTX+AT) and Total Parathyroidectomy (PTX)

Surgical steps are the same as for sPTX except that in this procedure, once the four hyperplastic glands are identified, all are resected[58-60,62-68]. When auto transplantation is performed (PTX +AT), the parathyroid chosen (usually the one less likely to have severe nodular hyperplasia) for reimplantation is morcelized into pieces of 1x1x1 mm. About 20 to 25 pieces (an overall weight of 50 to 100 mg) are implanted either in the ispilateral sterno-cleidomastoid muscle (orthotopic reimplant), or within the fore-arm brachioradialis muscle (avoiding the arm which has an artero-venous fistula) or even subcutaneously (heterotopic reimplant)[58,59,69,74]. The implantation pouches (usually more than one pouch is prepared to allow maximum growth of the graft) are closed using non-absorbable suture stitch and haemoclips are placed as reoperation is sometimes required[58,59,74]. PTX+AT has the advantage of reducing PTH levels avoiding permanent hypoparathyroidism, thus it would be chosen for patients scheduled for renal grafting[60,62,63]. PTX alone on the other hand would decrease and almost eliminate (unless the patient has ectopic parathyroid glands not removed during the operation) the risk for recurrence, but at the expense of developing adynamic bone disease. PTX produces favorable results in severely ill patients and all patients not eligible for transplantation[60,63,66-68].

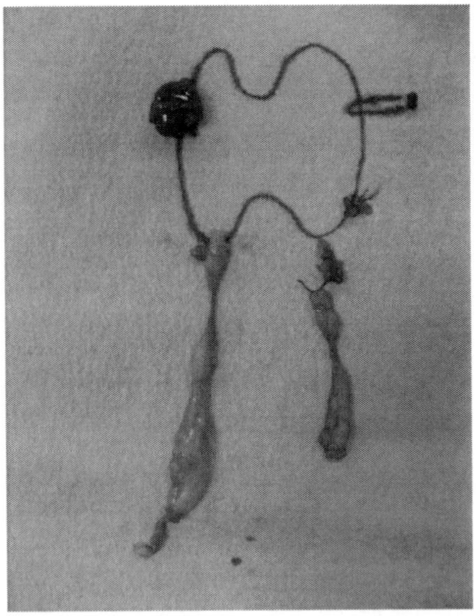

Figure 10.2. Outline of glands removed, with thymectomy. The left superior gland in this case has been used as the remnant as it would have been smaller and less nodular than the other glands.

Cryopreservation of Parathyroid Tissue and Delayed Transplantation

Cryopreservation is a well-described technique to preserve parathyroid tissue so as to be able to perform a late transplantation in patients operated on for renal hyperparathyroidism that then develop postoperative hypoparathyroidism[69]. Full viability of cryopreserved parathyroid tissue, differs in the literature ranging from 8% to 83%[69,70,77,79]. Recently, it has been proposed that cryopreservation might be done only in specialized centres, where the technique is standardized and always available, to maximize the effect of cryopreservation itself[70]. There are two factors affecting cryopreserved tissue function: A standardized technical procedure of cryopreservation and the mean time between initial resection and reimplantation[69,70]. The latter, actually, is linked with an inverse value to autograft function. The older the autograft has been stored the less it works[70] a year in storage is the maximum amount of time that parathyroid tissue can be reasonably stored for.

Parathyroid Aspiration to Confirm Parathyroid Origin

During operation for sHPT or tHPT the surgeon might have difficulty defining the tissue origin of all the nodules found, because patients with CRF often present with thyroid nodules[80]. Frozen section has been used to confirm the nature of the excised nodule. Nowadays, given the technical development of quick parathormone intra-operative measurement (IOPTH) some authors have described a standardized parathyroid aspiration technique to assess the origin of the tissue[80-82]. In situ or ex-vivo fine needle aspiration is made and the PTH level measured[81]. Overall accuracy of this technique reaches 95%, thus allowing the surgeon to avoid frozen section[80,82] and confirm the number and site of parathyroid glands found.

Intraoperative PTH Monitoring during Operation for Renal Hyperparathyroidism

IOPTH has been demonstrated as an important tool in determining the adequacy of parathyroid operation in primary hyperparathyroidism[55,80]. In a recent review of patients with renal hyperparathyroidism, the use of IOPTH has no impact on the surgical management of patients with sHPT, while it altered management in about 25% of patients with tHPT[83]. Some authors favor the use of IOPTH suggesting criteria of adequacy of resection based on PTH decrease[54,68,84]. Seehofer defined adequacy criteria to assess successful surgery[84]. A reduction of PTH 150 pg/ml or 30% of baseline is considered predictive for an optimal treatment[84]. However, the criterion for defining adequate resection differs among authors. Lorenz et al indicate a PTH value of 72 pg/ml at 20 minutes following PTX as indicative of curative resection, whereas Milas targeted the reduction of PTH to 200 pg/ml after sPTX[54,68]. However IOPTH monitoring is complicated in patients with CRF because of delayed renal clearance of PTH (delays of up to 60 minutes before IOPTH falls have been reported in the past), thus prolonging operative time in moderate to severely ill patients. Moreover the surgical goal is achieved when all four parathyroid glands are visualized. A delayed decrease in PTH levels after an appropriate resection would be a confounding element, resulting in a prolonged useless neck exploration. Optimal IOPTH criteria with reliable prediction of long-term success after resection are not yet established[68].

Post-Operative Complications

The mortality rate of parathyroidectomy in patients with sHPT and tHPT is usually low; overall mortality is up to 3.1% in different reports, with most of the deaths related to pre-existent medical conditions rather than the surgical procedure[4,54,63,67]. Permanent laryngeal nerve palsy has an incidence of 1%[4,54-57]. Transient hypocalcemia requiring oral supplementation, may be observed in up to 30% of patients[4,53,54,67]. Permanent hypoparathyroidism following sPTX or PTX is reported, but less frequently, ranging from 0 to 7%[5,54,77]. Additionally, patients requiring late cryopreserved parathyroid auto transplantation are reported to be up to 7%[4,54].

Which Surgical Approach?

The correct surgical strategy must be tailored to patients, each one of them is, by definition, unique and different. A rough categorization would divide patients with sHPT into two groups: those scheduled for a renal transplant and those who never will be transplanted. When patients are waiting for a graft and parathyroid surgery is mandatory, we would favor sPTX with cryopreservation of parathyroid tissue (when available) or PTX+AT. Normalization of renal function will remove all the biological conditions responsible for the development of sHPT and will keep the patient in a euparathyroid state. If PTX alone is performed, grafted patients will develop permanent hypoparathyroidism, and resultant hypercalciuria leading to a poor graft prognosis[54,57] and adynamic bone disease. In those patients not suitable for a renal transplant (i.e. lifelong hemodialysis), depending on surgeon experience and preference, all three surgical approaches may be used, keeping in mind the risk of reoperation for recurrence against those of adynamic bone disease which results after total parathyroidectomy without auto transplantation. The same strategies should be followed when dealing with tHPT; patients have a restored renal function thus sPTX (± cryopreservation) or PTX+AT would be the only surgical choices, to avoid a state of permanent hypoparathyroidism[53,55].

Effectiveness of Surgical Approaches: Persistent or Recurrent Hyperparathyroidism

Definition of "cure" for sHPT is a difficult point. Even though reduction in PTH is achieved after surgery, there is not a target level that defines the desirable level of PTH. Among different experiences the "ideal" level of PTH would range between 100 and 250 pg/ml following surgery[54,68,84]. Nevertheless, a rigid limit may not be applied to CRF patients, thus it is generally accepted a PTH level between 2 and 4 fold higher than the normal values[54]. PTH level has to be considered when followingup patients. Some of patients exhibit steady PTH values in the long-term whereas others demonstrate a slight but continuous increase in PTH leading to persistent/recurrent disease.

Persistent disease is defined as disease that develops within 6 months of the initial surgery. It is generally the result of a missed 5th or ectopic gland or an inadequate resection during the first operation[4,72,73,85-87]. The incidence of ersistence is higher for sPTX and PTX+AT in which a parathyroid remnant is left[85-87].

Recurrent disease is defined as disease that develops more than 6 months after initially successful surgery. It is obviously due to the permanent stimulus in CRF patients of residual parathyroid tissue; again it happens with a higher frequency after sPTX and PTX+AT[85-87]. Recurrences originate from: the remnant, the autograft, supernumerary glands or parathyromatosis[68,70,85-87].

Even though challenging, re-operation for recurrent/persistent disease is helped by localization studies. In fact MIBI scan, CT scan and MRI scan harbor a great sensitivity in this group of patients with theoretically a single gland disease, ranging from 85 up to 100% in different reports[4,56,57,87]. In case of ectopic mediastinal localization a minimally invasive approach (video-assisted thoracoscopic surgery, robot-assisted thoracoscopy, cervical mediastinoscopy) may be used to reduce morbidity and achieve a good post-operative outcome[88-91].

In patients previously treated with sPTX or PTX+AT, MIBI Scan may identify the source of persistence/recurrence within the neck or at the level of the transplanted parathyroid tissue. In the latter case, it is also possible to obtain a measurement of PTH level by venous sampling of both transplanted and not-transplanted arm, thus recognizing an eventual "arm" origin of recurrence (Casanova's Test)[58,75,76]. An eventual operation for graft-dependant recurrence (in case of heterotopic transplants) may be carried out under local anaesthesia 58,63,67].

In patients that have had an orthotopic transplant the scintigraphy uptake could depend either on a supernumerary parathyroid "left" in the neck, or the hyperfunctional graft [63,75,76].

Although many experiences are reported in the current literature, each claiming the superiority of one technique compared to the others, it is not possible to validate a standardized treatment for CRF patients with renal hyperparathyroidism.

In a randomized trial of 40 patients comparing sPTX to PTX+AT, the cure and recurrence rate achieved were better for those patients submitted to PTX+AT[56]. The incidence of persistent or recurrence disease widely differs in the literature, ranging from 2 to 80% for patients treated with sPTX or PTX+AT, whereas patients treated with PTX alone exhibit a lower rate (up to 4%)[53-65,85-87,92,93]. The risk of persistence/recurrence is directly proportional to post-operative PTH level. Thus patients with lower levels of PTH are less likely to need a second operation. Nevertheless some authors reported a successful reduction of PTH levels with sPTX and PTX+AT respectively of 96 and 100%[54,56].

On the other hand a wide number of publications recommend PTX as the procedure of choice in sHPT, claiming an extremely low recurrence rate (0 to 4%) in almost all the experiences[60-65]. Recently one publication, reporting a follow-up of more than 10 years in patients with sHPT treated with PTX, demonstrated recurrence in 7% of patients[63]. These large differences in surgical outcomes may be explained when analyzing different reports. Often the term "sub-total parathyroidectomy" referrs to those procedures in which a surgical exploration failed to identify all hyperplastic glands. Rather than a surgical exploration that does identify all 4 glands and selects the site and size of the remnant to leave behind. sPTX that has not found all the glands always recur leading to re-operation[60,64,93]. Reoperation increases the risk of complication, especially laryngeal nerve palsy[64].

Conclusion

Renal HPT derives from the disruption of calcium metabolism in patients with CRF. Such metabolic changes lead to the development of parathyroid hyperplasia and rise in PTH level. Consequently complications of hyperparathyroidism develop, worsening (sometimes critically as in calciphylaxis) the health of previously ill patients and eventually preventing a scheduled renal graft.

The optimal treatment for renal hyperparathyroidism is kidney transplantation. This corrects the calcium homeostasis removing the hyperplastic stimulus to the parathyroid glands. Alternatively a great part of patients may benefit from medical therapy that allows, a long and effective control of renal HPT in some. Nevertheless a small percentage of patients (up to 5%) require surgical removal of hyperplastic parathyroid glands. Different surgical options are available. The aim of parathyroidectomy is to control rather than eliminate PTH production but still, the type of surgery, must be tailored to each patient.

References

[1] Moe SM, Drueke TB. Management of secondary hyperparathyroidism: The importance and the challenge of controlling parathyroid hormone levels without elevating calcium, phosphorus and cacluim phosphorus product. *Am. J. Nephrol.* 2003; 23:369-379.

[2] de Francisco ALM. Secondary Hyperparathyroidism: Review of the Disease and Its Treatment. *Clin. Ther.* 2004;26(12):1976-1993.

[3] Breslau NA. Update on secondary forms of hyperparathyroidism. *Am. J. Med. Sci.* 1987;294:120-131.

[4] Pitt SC, Sippel RS, Chen H. Secondary and Tertiary Hyperparathyroidism. State of the Art, Surgical Management. *Surg. Clin. North Am.* 2009; 89(5): 1227-1239.

[5] Kebebew E, Duh QY, Clark OH. Tertiary Hyperparathyroidism; histologic patterns of disease and results of parathyroidectomy. *Arch. Surg.* 2004;139:974-977.

[6] Triponez F, Clark OH, Varenthergem Y et al. Surgical treatment of persistent hyperparathyroidism after renal transplantation. *Ann. Surg.* 2008; 248:18-30.

[7] Slatopolsky E, Delmez JA. Pathogenesis of secondary hyperparathyroidism. *Am. J. Kidney Dis.* 1994;23:229-236.

[8] Holick M. Vitamin D. Biosynthesis, metabolism and mode of action. In: DeGroot LJ (ed), Endocrinology, 2nd ed. Philadelphia, WB Saunders, 1989, p 902.

[9] Beckerman P, Silver J. Vitamin D and the parathyroid. *Am. J. Med. Sci.* 1999;317:363-369.

[10] Tokumoto M, Taniguchi M, Matsuo D et al. Parathyroid cell growth in patients with advanced secondary hyperparathyroidism: vitamin D receptors, calcium sensing receptor and cell cycle regulating factors. *Ther. Apher. Dial.* 2005;(9):S27-S34.

[11] Russel J, Lettieri D, Sherwood LM. Suppression by $1,25(OH)_2D_3$ of transcription of the pre-proparathyroid hormone gene. *Endocrinology* 1986;119:2864-2866.

[12] Akerstrom G, Rastad J, Ljunghall S et al. Cellular physiology and pathophysiology of the parathyroid glands. *World J. Surg.* 1991;15:672-680.

[13] Brown EM. Calcium receptor and regulation of parathyroid hormone secretion. *Rev. Endocr. Metab. Disord.* 2000;1:307-315.

[14] Slatopolsky E, Dusso A, Brown JA. The role of phosphorus in the development of secondary and tertiary hyperparathyroidism and parathyroid cell proliferation in chronic renal failure. *Am. J. Med. Sci.* 1999; 317:370-376.

[15] Rodriguez M. Direct effect of phosphate on parathyroid function. *Nephrol. Dial. Transplant.* 1999;(14):S1:70-72.

[16] Almaden Y, Hernandez A, Torregrossa V et al. High phosphate level directly stimulates parathyroid hormone secretion and synthesis by human parathyroid tissue in vitro. *J. Am. Soc. Nephrol.* 1998;9:1845-1952.

[17] Massry SG, Coburn JW, Lee DB et al. Skeletal resistance to parathyroid hormone in renal failure. Studies in 105 human subjects. *Ann. Intern Med.* 1973;78:357-364.

[18] Rosenblatt M, Kronenberg H, Potts J. Parathyroid hormone. Physiology, chemistry, biosynthesis, secretion, metabolism and mode of action. In: DeGroot LJ (ed), Endocrinology, 2nd ed. Philadelphia, WB Saunders, 1989, p 848.

[19] Felsenfeld AJ, Rodriguez M, Dunlay R, Llach F. A comparison of parathyroid gland function in haemodialysis patients with different forms of renal osteodystrophy. *Nephron Dial. Transplant.* 1991;6:244-251.

[20] Rahamimov R, Silver J. The molecular basis of secondary hyperparathyroidism in chronic renal failure. *Isr. J. Med. Sci.* 1994;30(1):26-31.

[21] Salusky IB, Goodman WG. Renal ostedystrophy in dialyzed children. *Miner. Electrolyte Metab.* 1991;17:273-280.

[22] Slatopolsky E, Brown JA, Dusso A. Pathogenesis of secondary hyperparathyroidism. *Kidney Int Suppl.* 1999;73:S14-S19.

[23] Hruska K: Pathophysiology of renal osteodystrophy. *Pediatr. Nephrol.* 2000;14:636–640.

[24] Gerakis A, Hadjiakis D, Kokkinakis E, et al. Correlation of bone mineral density with the histological finding of renal osteodystrophy in patients on haemodialysis. *J. Nephron.* 2000;13:437-443.

[25] Spasovsky GB, Bervoets AR, Behets GJ et al. Spectrum of renal bone disease in end-stage renal failure patients not yet in dialysis. *Nephron. Dial. Transplant.* 2003;18:1159-1166.

[26] Chazan JA, Libbey NP, London MR et al. The clinical spectrum of renal osteo-dystrophy in 57 chronic haemodialysis patients: A correlation between biochemical parameters and bone pathology findings. *Nephrol.* 1991;35(2):78-85..

[27] Monier-Faugere MC, Malluche HH. Trends in renal osteodystrophy: a survey from 1983 and 1995 in a total of 2248 patients.*Nephron Dial. Transplant,* 1996;11(S3):111-120.

[28] Timmins S, Hibbert M. Images in Clinical Medicine. Metastatic pulmonary calcification. *N. Eng. J. Med.* 2010 Dec;363(26):2547.

[29] Tarrass F, Benjelloun M, Zamd M et al. Heart valve calcification in patients with end stage renal disease: analysis for risk factors. *Nephrology*, (Carlton) 2006 Dec; 11(6):494-496.

[30] Cowlam TE, Bucknall TE. Cutaneous ectopic breast calcification in a haemodialysis patient. *Breast,* 2003 Oct;12(5):342-344.

[31] Foley RN. Clinical epidemiology of cardiac disease in dialysis patients: left ventricular hypertrophy, ischemic heart disease and cardiac failure. *Semin. Dial.* 2003;16:111-117.

[32] Floegel I, Klein A, Langmann G. Metastatic schlerochoroidal calcification involving the fovea. *Retina*, 2002 Aug;22(4):503-505.

[33] Klaassen-Broekema N, van Bijsterveld OP. Red eyes in renal failure. *Br. J. Ophthalmol.* 1992 May;76(5):268-71.

[34] Aktaş Z, Ozdek S, Asli Dinç U, Akyürek N, Atalay V, Güz G, Hasanreisoglu B. Alterations in ocular surface and corneal thickness in relation to metabolic control in patients with chronic renal failure. *Nephrology* (Carlton). 2007 Aug;12(4):380-5.

[35] Toorians AW, Jansen E, Laan E et al. Chronic renal failure and sexual functioning: clinical status versus objectively assessed sexual response. *Nephron. Dial. Transplant.* 1997;12:2654-2663.

[36] Neves KR, Graciolli FG, dos Reis LM et al. Vascular calcification: contribution of parathyroid hormone in renal failure. Kidney Int 2007 Jun;71(12):1262-1270.

[37] Rostand SG, Drueke TB. Parathyroid hormone, vitamin D and cardiovascular disease in chronic renal failure. Kidney Int 1999;56:383-392.

[38] London GM, De Vernejoul MC, Fabiani F, et al. Secondary hyperparathyroidism and cardiac hypertrophy in haemodialysis patients. Kidney Int 1987;32(6):900-907..

[39] Pizzarelli F,Fabrizi F, Postorino M et al. Parathyroidectomy and blood pressure in hemodialysis patients. *Nephron*, 1993;63:384-389.

[40] Carmichael AJ, McHugh MM, Martin AM, Farrow M. Serological markers of renal itch in patients receiving long term haemodialysis. *Br. Med. J.* (Clin Res Ed). 1988; 296:1575.

[41] Chou FF, Ho JC, Huang SC, Scheen-Chen SM. A study on pruritus after parathyroidectomy for secondary hyperparathyroidism. *J. Am. Coll. Surg.* 2000;190:65-70.

[42] Massry SG. Pathogenesis of the anemia in uremia: Role of secondary hyperparathyroidism. Kidney Int Suppl 1983;16:S204-S207.

[43] Levin A, Metha RL, Goldstein GB. Mathematical formulation to help identify the patient at risk of ischemic tissue necrosis-A potentially lethal complication of chronic renal failure. Iol on parathyroid function and on bone remodeling in secondary hyperparathyroidism. *Nephron Dial. Am. J. Nephrol.* 1993;13:448-453.

[44] Roe SM, Graham LD, Brock WB, Barker DE. Calciphylaxis. Early recognition and management. *Am. Surg.* 1994;60(2):81-86.

[45] Duh QY, Lim RC, Clark OH. Calciphylaxis in secondary hyperparathyroidism. Diagnosis and parathyroidectomy. *Arch. Surg.* 1991;126: 1213-1219.

[46] National Kidney Foundation: K/DOQI clinical practice guidelines for bone metabolism and disease in chronic kidney disease. *Am. J. Kidney Dis.* 2003; 42:S1-S202.

[47] Indridason OS, Quarles LD, for the Durham Rean Osteodystrophy Study Group. Comparison of treatments for mild secondary hyperparathyroidism in hemodialysis patients. Kidney Int 2000;57:282-292.

[48] Costa AF, dos Reis LM, RIbeiro MC, et al. Effects of calcitriol on parathyroid function and on bone remodelling in secondary hyperparathyroidism. *Blood Purif.* 1996;14:234-241.

[49] Lindberg JS, Culleton B, Wong G et al. Cinacalcet HCL, an Oral Calcimimetic Agent for the Treatment of Secondary Hyperparathyroidism in Hemodialysis and Peritoneal Dialysis: A Randomized Double-Blind, Multicenter Study. *J. Am. Soc. Nephrol.* 2005; 16:800-807.

[50] Block GA, Martin KJ, de Francisco AL et al. Cinacalcet for secondary hyperparathyroidism in patients receiving hemodialysis. *N. Eng. J. Med.* 2004;350:1516-1525.

[51] Kerby JD, Rue LW, Blair H, Hudson S, Sellers MT, Diethelm AG. Operative treatment of tertiary hyperparathyroidism: a single centre experience. *Ann. Surg.* 1998;227 (6):878-886.

[52] Triponez F, Kebebew E, Dosseh D, Duh QY, Hazzan M, Noel C, Chertow GM, Wambergue F, Fleury D, Lemaitre V, Proye C, Clark OH. Less-than-subtotal parathyroidectomy increases the risk of persistent/recurrent hyperparathyroidism after renal transplantation. *Surgery,* 2006; 140(6):990-997.

[53] Traindl O, Langle F, Reading S, et al. Secondary hyperparathyroidism and acute tubular necrosis following renal transplantation. Nephrol Dial Transplant 1993;8(2):173-176.Milas M, Weber C. Near-total parathyroidectomy is beneficial for patients with secondary and tertiary hyperparathyroidism. *Surgery*, 2004;136:1252-1260.

[54] Milas M, Weber C. Near-total parathyroidectomy is beneficial for patients with secondary and tertiary hyperparathyroidism. *Surgery*, 2004;136:1252-1260.

[55] Adler JT, Sippel RS, Chen HNew Trends in Parathyroid Surgery. *Curr. Probl. Surg.* 2010;(12): 958-1017.

[56] Mihai R, Simon D, Hellman P. Imaging for primary hyperparathyroidism – an evidence-based analysis. *Langenbecks Arch. Surg.* 2009;394(5):765-784.

[57] Gasparri G, Camandona M, Bertoldo U et al. The usefulness of preoperative dual-phase 99mTc MIBI-scintigraphy and IO-PTH assay in the treatment of secondary and tertiary hyperparathyroidism. *Ann. Surg.* 2009;250(6):868-871.

[58] Niederle B. Secondary parathyroid hyperplasia surgical strategy: subtotal or total parathyroidectomy with autograft. *Acta Chir. Austriaca.* 1996;124:4-8.

[59] Rothmund M, Wagner PK, Schark C. Subtotal parathyroidectomy *versus* total parathyroidectomy and auto transplantation for secondary hyperparathyroidism: a randomized trial. *World J. Surg.* 1991;15:745-750.

[60] Nicholson ML, Veitch PS, Feehally J. Parathyroidectomy in chronic renal failure: comparison of three operative strategies. *J. R. Coll. Surg.* Edinb.1996;41:382-387.

[61] Shen WT, Kebebew E, Suh I, Duh QY, Clark OH. Two hundred and two consecutive operation for secondary hyperparathyroidism: has medical management changed the profiles of patients requiring parathyroidectomy? *Surgery* 2009; 146 (2):296-299.

[62] Niederle B, Roka R, BrennanMF. The transplantation of parathyroid tissue in man: development, indications, technique and results. *Endocr. Rev.* 1982;3:245-279.

[63] Schlosser K, Veit JA, Witte S, Férnandez ED, Victor N, Knaebel HP et al. Comparison of total parathyroidectomy without transplantation and without thymectomy versus total parathyroidectomy with auto transplantation and with thymectomy for secondary hyperparathyroidism: TOPAR PILOT-Trial. Trials 2007;8:22.

[64] Tominaga Y, Matsuoka S, Sato T. Surgical indications and procedures of parathyroidectomy in patients with chronic kidney disease. *Ther. Apher. Dial.* 2005; 9:44-47.

[65] Shih ML, Duh QY, Hsieh CB, Lin SH, Wu HS, Chu PL et al. Total parathyroidectomy without auto transplantation for secondary hyperparathyroidism. *World J. Surg.* 2009;33:248-254.

[66] Puccini M, Carpi A, Cupisti A, Caprioli R, Iacconi P et al. Total parathyroidectomy without auto transplantation for the treatment of secondary hyperparathyroidism associated with chronic kidney disease: clinical and laboratori long-term follow-up. *Biomed. Pharmacother.* 2010;64(5):359-362.

[67] Coulston JE, Egan R, Willis E, Morgan JD. Total parathyroidectomy without auto transplantation for renal hyperparathyroidism. *Br. J. Surg.* 2010;97:1674-1679.

[68] Lorenz K, Ukkat J, Sekulla C, Gimm O, Brauckhoff M, Dralle H. Total parathyroid-ectomy without auto transplantation for renal hyperparathyroidism: Experience with a qPTH-controlled Protocol. *World J. Surg.* 2006; 30:743-751.

[69] Cohen MS, Dillye WG, Wells SA Jr, Moley JF, Doherty GM et al. Long-term functionality of cryopreserved parathyroid autografts: A 13-year prospective analysis. *Surgery* 2005;138(6):1033-1041.

[70] Borot S, Lapierre V, Carnaille B, Goudet P, Penformis A. Results of cryopreserved parathyroid autografts: A retrospective multicenter study. *Surgery* 2010; 147(4):529-535.

[71] Akerstrom G, Rudberg C, GrimeliusL et al. Recurrent hyperparathyroidism due to preoperative seeding of neoplastic or hyperplastic parathyroid tissue. Case report. *Acta Chir. Scand.* 1988;154:549-552.

[72] Cattan P, Halimi B, Aidan K et al. Reoperation for secondary uremic hyperpara-thyroidism: are tecnical difficulties influenced by initial surgical procedures? *Surgery* 2000;127(5):620-625.

[73] Pattou FN, Pellissier LC, Nöel C, Wambergue F, Huglo DG, Proye CA. Supernumerary parathyroid glands: frequency and surgical significance in the treatment of renal hyperparathyroidism. *World J. Surg.* 2000;24:1330-1334.

[74] Monchik JM, Bendinelli C, Passero MA Jr, Roggin KK. Subcutaneous forearm transplantation of autologous parathyroid tissue in patients with renal hyperpara-thyroidism. *Surgery* 1999; 126(6): 1152-1158.

[75] Walgenbach S, Hommel G, Juginger T. Prospective evaluation of parathyroid graft function after total parathyroidectomy and heterotopic transplantation in renal hyperparathyroidism by bilateral determination of intact parathormone in cubital venous blood. *World J. Surg.* 1998;22:93-97.

[76] Casanova D, Sarfati E, De Francisco A et al. Secondary hyperparathyroidism: diagnosis of site of recurrence. *World J. Surg.* 1991;15:546-549.

[77] Wells SA Jr, Farndon JR, Dale JK et al. Long-term evaluation of patients with primary parathyroid hyperplasia managed by total parathyroidectomy and heterotopic transplantation. *Ann. Surg.* 1980; 192:451-458.

[78] Saxe AW, Spiegel AM, Marx SJ, Brennan MF. Deferred parathyroid autografts with cryopreserved tissue after reoperative parathyroid surgery. *Arch. Surg.* 1982;117:538-543.

[79] Herrera M, Grant C, van Heerden JA, Fitzpatrick LA. Parathyroid auto transplantation. *Arch. Surg.* 1992;127:825-829; discussion 829-830.

[80] Iacobone M, Scarpa M, Lumachi F, Favia G. Are frozen section useful and cost-effective in the era of intraoperative qPTH assay? *Surgery*, 2005; 138(6):1159-1165.

[81] Lo CY, Chan WF, Leung P, Luk JM. Applicability of Tissue Aspirate for Quick Parathyroid Hormone Assay to Confirm Parathyroid Tissue Identity During Parathyroidectomy for Primary Hyperparathyroidism. *Arch. Surg.* 2005;140:146-149.

[82] Horanyi J, Duffek L, Szlavik R, Takacs I et al. Intraoperative Determination of PTH Concentrations in Fine Needle Tissue Aspirates to Identify Parathyroid Tissue During Parathyroidectomy. *World J. Surg.* 2010; 34(3): 538-543.

[83] Pitt SC, Panneerselvan R, Chen H et al. Secondary and tertiary hyperparathyroidism: the utility of ioPTH monitoring. *World J. Surg.* 2010;34:343-349.

[84] Seehofer D, Rayes N, Klupp J et al. Predictive value of intact parathyroid hormone measurement during surgery for renal hyperparathyroidism. *Langenbecks Arch. Surg.* 2005; 390(3):222-229.

[85] Henry JF, Denizot A, Audiffret J et al. Results of reoperations for persistent or recurrent secondary hyperparathyroidism in hemodialysis patients. *World J. surg.* 1990;14:303-307.

[86] Skinner K, Zuckerbaun L. Recurrent secondary hyperparathyroidism. An argument for total parathyroidectomy. *Arch. Surg.* 1996;131:724-727.

[87] Gasparri G, Camandona M, Abbona GC, Papotti M, Jeantet A, Radice E, Mullineris B, Dei Poli M. Secondary and Tertiary Hyperparathyroidism: Cases of Recurrent Disease after 446 Parathyroidectomies. *Ann. Surg.* 2001; 233(1):65-69.

[88] Inabnet WB, Chu CA. Transcervical endoscopic-assisted mediastinal parathyroid-ectomy with intraoperative parathyroid hormone monitoring. Surg. Endosc. 2003 Oct;17(10):1678.

[89] Ismail M, Maza S, Swierzy M, Tsilimparis N, Rogalla P, Sandrock D, Rückert RI, Müller JM, Rückert JC. Resection of ectopic mediastinal parathyroid glands with the da Vinci robotic system. *Br. J. Surg.* 2010;97(3):337-43.

[90] Iacobone M, Mondi I, Viel G, Citton M, Tropea S, Frego M, Favia G. The results of surgery for mediastinal parathyroid tumors: a comparative study of 63 patients. *Langenbecks Arch. Surg.* 2010;395(7):947-953.

[91] Alesina PF, Moka D, Mahlstedt J, Walz MK. Thoracoscopic Removal of Mediastinal Hyperfunctoning Parathyroid Glands: Personal Experience and Review of the Literature. *World J. Surg.* 2008:32:224-231. Review

[92] Kenstenbaum B, Andress DL, Schwarz SM et al. Survival following parathyroidectomy among United States dialysis patients. Kidney Int 2004;66:2010-2016.

[93] Stracke S, Jehle PM, Sturm D, Schoenberg MH, Widmaier U, berger H et al. Clinical course after total parathyroidectomy in patients with end-stage renal failure. *Am. J. Kidney Dis.* 1999; 33:304-311.

In: Parathyroid: Anatomy, Functions and Disorders
Editor: James Kirkby-Bott
ISBN: 978-1-62100-765-4

Chapter XI

Predictors of Ectopic Parathyroid Gland Location and Imaging Failure in Patients with Persistent or Recurrent Hyperparathyroidism

Haridimos Markogiannakis, Bill Fleming, and James Kirkby-Bott
[1] Dept Surgery, Hippokration Hospital, Athens, Greece
[2] Endocrine Surgical Unit, Western Health, Melbourne, Victoria, Australia
Kingston Hospital, Kingston-upon-Thames, Surrey, UK

Abstract

Re-operation for persistent or recurrent hyperparathyroidism can present significant challenges. Predictive factors of ectopic parathyroid gland location and failure of imaging in patients with persistent or recurrent hyperparathyroidism are reviewed. Ectopic gland location is frequent in re-operative disease with a reported incidence of 23-77%. Multivariate analysis identified secondary and persistent disease as predictors of ectopic glands (all ectopic locations).

Renal HPT patients were more prone to have ectopic glands while those with concomitant thyroid pathology less likely to have mediastinal glands. Secondary disease and high number of previously removed glands were associated with a thymic location. Ultrasound failure is higher in ectopic glands, secondary HPT predicts sestamibi failure and ectopic location was a predictor of combined ultrasound and sestamibi failure. Combined selective venous sampling and parathyroid angiography have an accuracy rate of 95%.

Meticulous pre-operative investigation is crucial for successful treatment of patients with persistent and recurrent hyperparathyroidism. The identified factors are useful for interpreting imaging results and planning surgical strategy in re-operations and they give insight into reasons for failure that help define a strategy when dealing with difficult initial operations. Such factors are very useful for interpreting imaging results and planning operative strategy in this group of patients.

Introduction

Re-operation for persistent or recurrent hyperparathyroidism (HPT) can present significant challenges for the endocrine surgeon. Fortunately, persistent or recurrent HPT is uncommon with initial surgery being an effective treatment for both primary and secondary disease with a 90-98% success rate.[1-10] Once a biochemical diagnosis of persistent or recurrent disease is confirmed, a thorough evaluation of previous radiology, operative and pathology findings is essential. Further imaging studies for the localization of the abnormal parathyroid gland/s and knowledge of their potential location are crucial for offering the highest likelihood of cure while minimizing the risk of complications in re-operative surgery.[10-20] Predictive factors of ectopic parathyroid gland location and failure of imaging studies in patients with persistent or recurrent HPT are of the utmost importance for interpreting imaging results and planning operative strategy.

Several studies have investigated the value of imaging modalities in previously un-operated HPT patients, fewer, in persistent or recurrent cases, and the vast majority of them have evaluated a limited number of parameters using only univariate analysis.

In this chapter we have used data collected by the authors to show how meticulous pre-operative investigation and the use of parathyroid angiography and venous sampling can improve outcomes and correlated this with the literature. It is the authors opinion that secondary disease is best dealt with by an adequate first operation with marking of remnant glands and a detailed operative report to assist in the often predictable need for re-operation in cases of multigland primary HPT and secondary HPT using operative strategies outlined in chapters 5 and 10. The anatomy of parathyroids and the embryological explanation for variation in positions is discussed in chapter 1.

Outcomes of Primary Surgery

Most patients are cured at the initial operation for hyperparathyroid disease by an experienced endocrine surgeon.[1-10,16,21-23] Despite this success rate, persistent and recurrent HPT remain challenging clinical entities. The factors that commonly contribute to treatment failure can be categorized as the initial surgical procedure and the surgeons response to anatomic variability, and the biology of the disease process.[3-9,13-15,18, 19,22,24,25] An understanding of these factors can prevent persistence and recurrence and plays an integral role in planning re-operation. Re-operative parathyroid surgery exposes patients to a higher risk of complications and increases surgical challenges and should only be undertaken by an experienced endocrine surgeon in a specialist endocrine centre.[3,4,8,10,17-19,23,25] Cure rate in repeat parathyroid surgery in the literature ranges between 81.8% and 100% [5-23,25-29]. Transient and permanent nerve palsy have been reported from 0% to 8.7% and 0% to 7.9%, respectively[5,7-10,13,17-20,22,23,25-28]. These results noted in experienced hands in endocrine surgical centres indicate that the historical opinion that re-operation is associated with more complications and fewer cures compared to initial surgery may have been exaggerated by results of inexperienced endocrine surgeons, and may be no longer true in the era of specialist endocrine surgery and meticulous preoperative localisation [3,5-7,10,11,13,18-20,23,26,27]. A significant percentage of persistent primary HPT is due to an unidentified orthotopic cervical gland. Mis-labelling of superior and inferior parathyroids based on location in neck rather than relationship with the recurrent laryngeal nerve can cause confusion in re-operations undertaken without adequate localisation before surgery. Strategies for dealing with anticipated recurrence in secondary HPT and ways to minimise persistence are covered in chapter 10 on secondary and tertiary HPT.

Ectopic Parathyroid Glands

Ectopic location is frequent in studies for re-operative parathyroid surgery ranging between 23.8% and 77.4% [6-9,13,16-20,22-29]. Multivariate analysis identifies persistent primary and secondary HPT as predictors of ectopic location (table 11.1). Patients with secondary HPT and persistent primary HPT had a 7.9 and 2.9 times greater odds of ectopic glands than those with primary adenoma and recurrent disease, respectively in a recent study by the chapter authors. In accordance with our result, others have reported that the abnormal glands were ectopic in 80% of cases re-operated for persistent secondary HPT in contrast to 46.6% of patients with recurrent secondary disease [7,28] . In addition, it has been noted that 60% of the glands were ectopic in patients with persistent primary HPT compared to 36.3% in recurrent HPT cases [13]. It has also observed that 64% of secondary HPT patients had ectopic glands as opposed to 49% of primary cases; however, this difference was not statistically significant in the univariate analysis [13]. A high index of suspicion of an ectopic location of the abnormal parathyroid gland is therefore needed in patients under going surgery for persistent or secondary HPT.

Table 1. Comparison between the Ectopic and Orthotopic group (univariate analysis)

VARIABLE	ECTOPIC GROUP (n=29)	ORTHOTOPIC GROUP (n=51)	p
Age (years)[1]	56.3±12.7	59.4±14.6	0.31
Sex (Female / Male)[2]	21 (72.4%) / 8 (27.6%)	35 (68.6%) / 16 (31.4%)	0.6
Number of previous operations for HPT[2]			0.3
One	22 (75.8%)	43 (84.3%)	
Two	7 (24.2%)	8 (15.7%)	
Number of previously removed glands[3]	1 (1)	1 (1)	0.8
Type of HPT[2]			0.09
Persistent	24 (82.7%)	33 (64.7%)	
Recurrent	5 (17.3%)	18 (35.3%)	
Etiology[2]			0.003
Parathyroid adenoma	19 (65.5%)	43 (84.3%)	
Primary hyperplasia	3 (10.3%)	6 (11.7%)	
Secondary hyperplasia	7 (24.2%)	2 (4%)	
Previous thyroid surgery[2]	6 (20.6%)	6 (11.7%)	0.26
Concomitant thyroid pathology[2]	5 (17.2%)	9 (17.6%)	0.96
Pre-operative calcium (mmol/L)[1]	2.88±0.22	2.87±0.16	0.78
Pre-operative PTH (pmol/L)[3]	50 (20)	30 (10)	0.19
Parathyroid gland weight (gr)[3]	830 (135)	610 (240)	0.09

[1] Values are expressed as mean±SD (standard deviation).
[2] Values are presented as number of patients and percentage (parenthesis).
[3] Values are expressed as median and inter-quartile range (in parenthesis).

Predictors of Ectopic Location

The abnormal glands are often positioned in the mediastinum a finding that is consistent among studies (22%-66.3%) [7-9,13,16-19,22,24-29]. In multivariate analysis, secondary HPT patients were found to be more prone to have mediastinal glands in comparison to patients with a concomitant thyroid multi-nodular goitre. Unsurprisingly a higher proportion of patients with mediastinal glands had undergone two previous operations for HPT than the non-mediastinal group. In agreement with our finding for patients that had failed surgery for secondary HPT, Hibi *et al.* reported that 37% of the responsible glands were mediastinal in cases re-operated for persistent/recurrent secondary HPT[7]. On the contrary, the higher likelihood of re-operative HPT patients with concomitant multi-nodular goitre having a cervical location of the abnormal gland/s demonstrated by the authors has not been investigated before.

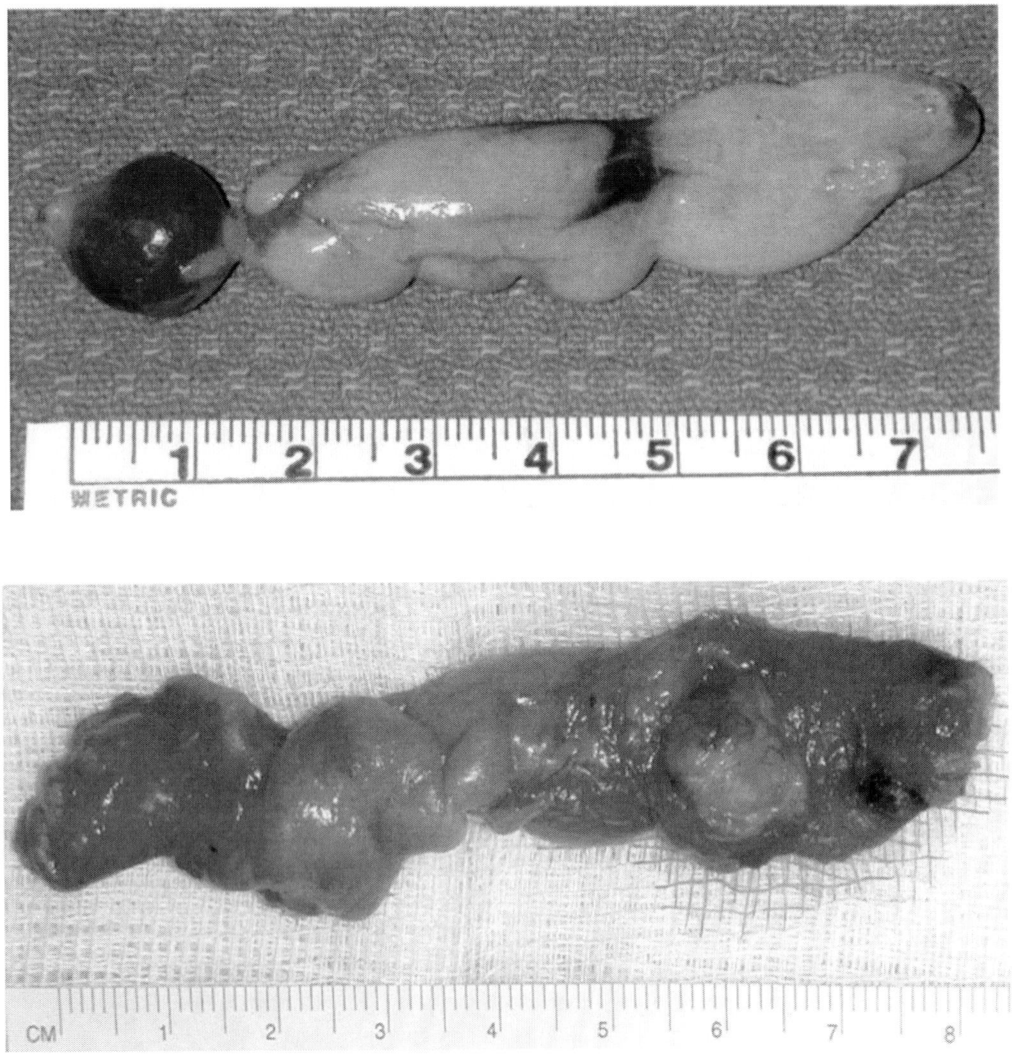

Figure 11.1. and 11.2. show thymic parathyroid glands.

Table 2. Comparison between Thymic group and Non-thymic group (univariate analysis)

VARIABLE	THYMIC GROUP (n=17)	NON-THYMIC GROUP (n=63)	p
Age (years)[1]	60.3±8.8	57.6±15.2	0.43
Sex (Female / Male)[2]	12 (70.6%) / 5 (29.4%)	44 (69.8%) / 19 (30.2%)	0.86
Number of previous operations for HPT[2]			0.22
One	12 (70.6%)	53 (84.1%)	
Two	5 (29.4%)	10 (15.9%)	
Number of previously removed glands[3]	2 (1)	1 (1)	0.005
Type of HPT[2]			0.91
Persistent	12 (70.6%)	45 (71.4%)	
Recurrent	5 (29.4%)	18 (28.6%)	
Etiology[2]			0.001
Parathyroid adenoma	7 (41.1%)	55 (87.3%)	
Primary hyperplasia	3 (17.8%)	6 (9.5%)	
Secondary hyperplasia	7 (41.1%)	2 (3.2%)	
Previous thyroid surgery[2]	3 (17.6%)	9 (14.3%)	0.79
Concomitant thyroid pathology[2]	1 (5.8%)	13 (20.6%)	0.12
Pre-operative calcium (mmol/L)[1]	2.83±0.25	2.88±0.23	0.37
Pre-operative PTH (pmol/L)[3]	49 (13)	34 (8)	0.21
Parathyroid gland weight (gr)[3]	750 (270)	665 (190)	0.47

[1]Values are expressed as mean±SD (standard deviation).
[2]Values are presented as number of patients and percentage (parenthesis).
[3]Values are expressed as median and inter-quartile range (in parenthesis).

Our results indicate that surgeons should be highly suspicious of mediastinal glands in re-operative secondary HPT cases while a thorough exploration of all potential, orthotopic or ectopic, cervical locations is likely to yield the elusive tumor in patients with a multi-nodular goitre. Since a substantial portion of mediastinal glands are intra-thymic, cervical thymectomy can frequently result in successful retrieval of the mediastinal tumor and should be performed before mediastinal exploration (figures 11.1 and 11.2). The latter should be reserved for patients with mediastinal pathology, confirmed by imaging, when no parathyroid gland is found in the resected thymus gland (figure 11.3). Thymic location is common with an incidence of 12.8%-45% in published series [6-9,13,16-19,22,25,28]. Secondary HPT and the number of previously removed glands were identified as predictors of thymic parathyroid glands (table 11.2). Patients with secondary HPT had 15.1 times greater odds for thymic glands than those with a primary adenoma and 20% of the abnormal glands in patients re-operated for persistent or recurrent secondary HPT were thymic[7]. Univariate analysis has also revealed an association of thymic location with primary HPT due to hyperplasia rather than adenoma, as one might expect from the correlation with secondary HPT. Because an ectopic or supernumerary gland is often located in the thymus, routine bilateral thymectomy is advocated to avoid or reduce the risk of persistence or recurrence in previously unoperated secondary failure patients and in re-operations for primary or secondary HPT [7,9,22]. The results of this study also underscore the high likelihood of thymic location of the hyper-functioning gland/s in re-operative secondary HPT cases and, additionally, in all re-operative patients who had two or more glands previously removed. The majority of thymic tumors can be removed by delivering the thymus into the neck, using gentle, steady upward traction on the upper tongue of the thymus. However, a few are situated deep in the mediastinum and are inaccessible to retrieval from the neck. These lesions require mediastinal exploration for their removal. This can be achieved with manubriotomy[30] or thoroscopic techniques[31].

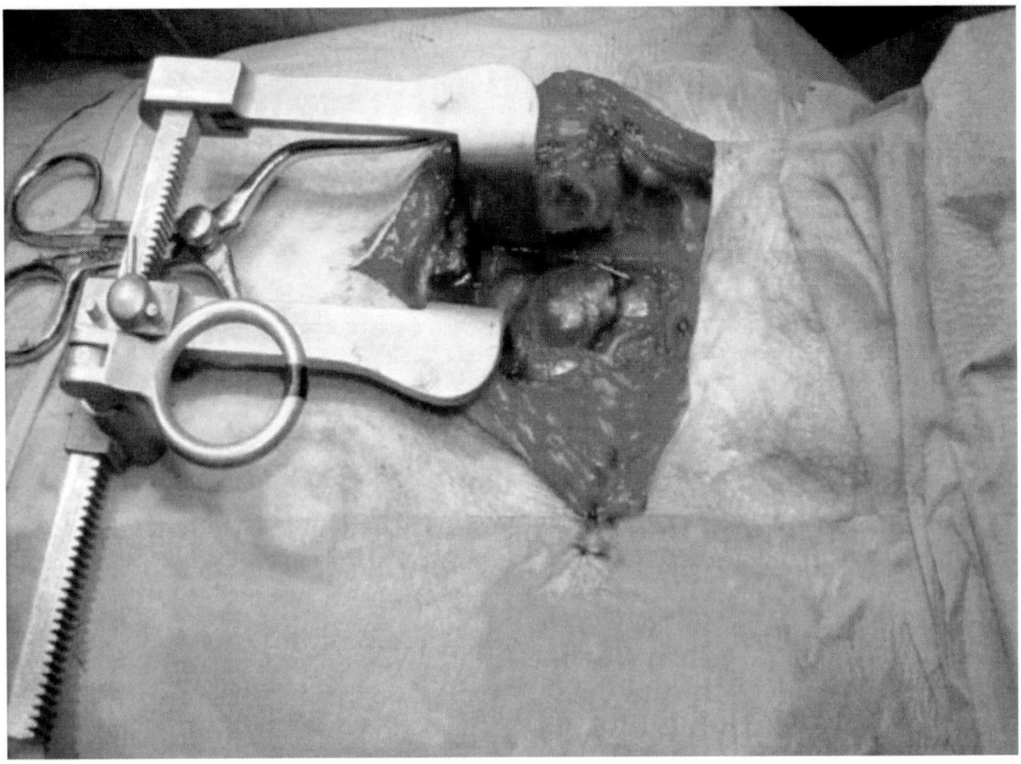

Figure 11.3. shows a parathyroid found outside the thymus glands via a manubriotomy. A Kocher incision had been performed first and thymectomy undertaken with no gland retrieved. At this point manubriotomy was undertaken.

Imaging in Redo Parathyroid Surgery

Previous reports agree that US and MIBI are adequate for localisation in 50%-80% of the patients when used as a single modality; while combined evaluation of both methods yields an accuracy of 80%-93.5% in re-operative series [7,8,10,11,13,14,18-20,23,26-29,32]. Which compares favourably with earlier reports of 70-100% accuracy for selective venous sampling or Parathyroid angiography [11,13-20,22,24,27].

Table 3. Risk factors of failure of both ultrasound and sestamibi (univariate analysis)

VARIABLE	SUCCESS GROUP (n=69)	FAILURE GROUP (n=11)	p
Age (years)[1]	56.3±18.6	58.8±11.5	0.25
Sex (Female / Male)[2]	48 (69.6%) / 21 (30.4%)	8 (72.8%) / 3 (27.2%)	0.54
Number of previous operations for HPT[2]			0.92
One	56 (81.1%)	9 (81.9%)	
Two	13 (18.9%)	2 (18.1%)	
Number of previously removed glands[3]	1 (1)	1 (1)	0.8
Type of HPT[2]			0.56
Persistent	50 (72.5%)	7 (63.7%)	
Recurrent	19 (27.5%)	4 (36.3%)	
Etiology[2]			0.07
Parathyroid adenoma	56 (81.2%)	6 (54.7%)	
Primary hyperplasia	7 (10.1%)	2 (18.1%)	
Secondary hyperplasia	6 (8.7%)	3 (27.2%)	
Previous thyroid surgery[2]	10 (14.5%)	2 (18.1%)	0.74
Concomitant thyroid pathology[2]	12 (17.4%)	2 (18.1%)	0.94
Pre-operative calcium (mmol/L)[1]	2.89±0.17	2.85±0.2	0.22
Pre-operative PTH (pmol/L)[3]	44 (12)	42 (14)	0.94
Parathyroid gland weight (gr)[3]	820 (170)	640 (210)	0.35
Gland location[2]			0.003
Ectopic	21 (30.4%)	8 (72.8%)	
Orthotopic	48 (69.6%)	3 (27.2%)	

[1]Values are expressed as mean±SD (standard deviation).
[2]Values are presented as number of patients and percentage (parenthesis).
[3]Values are expressed as median and inter-quartile range (in parenthesis).

However, combined venous sampling and parathyroid angiography were highly successful in localisation of the elusive tumor with an accuracy of 94.1%, a result that is consistent with other series [10]. As ultrasound and sestamibi are less reliable in reoperative disease (table 11.3), venous sampling and parathyroid angiography are very valuable and, thus, warranted in re-operative disease, particularly when US and Sestamibi fail [4,11,13,15-20,24,27].

Ultrasound in Persistent Hyperparathyroidism

Ectopic parathyroid gland location has been identified as an independent predictor of US failure. Patients with ectopic glands had 11.9 times higher odds of non-successful localization by US than patients with orthotopic glands. Although this result is most likely attributed to the fact that the majority (78.8%) of ectopic glands in our study were in the mediastinum, a location that can not be accurately evaluated by sonography due to the overlying bony thoracic cage,[17,29] US failure may also often occur in atypically localized cervical glands [17,29]. In a meta-analysis of 17 publications regarding preoperative US in patients submitted to re-operative parathyroid surgery the number of true positive results was markedly higher in cases with orthotopic cervical location of the abnormal glands [17]. It has been demonstrated that only 50% of glands are localised with US with a 23% accuracy rate[7, 28]. It has been observed that among 22 undetected tumors, 3 were orthotopic, 4 retro-tracheal/retro-esophageal and one intra-thyroidal while US also failed in all 14 mediastinal glands [29]

None of the other analyzed parameters, including gland weight, hyperplasia, number of prior operations for HPT and previous thyroidectomy, affected the accuracy of US in our study, a result that is similar to that of other investigators [29]. Two studies of previously unoperated primary HPT patients, using only univariate analysis, found a positive correlation between parathyroid adenoma weight and true-positive US results [33,34]. Thyroid nodularity was more common in patients with false-positive or false-negative US than in the total population of 116 initial and 26 re-operative cases[32] and US sensitivity decreased from 100% in patients without nodules to 84% in those with thyroid nodules[33]. In the authors experience, patients with concomitant thyroid multi-nodular goitre were also more common in those whom ultrasound did not localise the adenoma. The overall evidence suggests that a high index of suspicion for ectopic location is required in patients with a negative US study, but that in the presence of a multinodular goitre a cervical location is still likely. This suspicion should be even higher in cases of negative US results and persistent or secondary HPT, as shown by the multivariate analysis for predictors of ectopic location in our study.

Sestamibi in Persistent Hyperparathyroidism

Multivariate analysis, in our series for this chapter, has identified secondary HPT as the sole predictor of MIBI failure. Patients with renal hyperplasia had 8.7 greater odds of a non-successful MIBI result compared to cases with an adenoma. Our result regarding MIBI failure in renal hyperplasia is in keeping with other studies of HPT patients before initial surgery [21,35,36] or reoperation[37]. Although primary hyperplasia was associated with failure in univariate analysis, it was not found to be an independent predictor of MIBI failure in multivariate analysis. However, it is generally thought that MIBI is less sensitive in para-thyroid hyperplasia. One study found that localization of the pathologic gland by MIBI was correct in all re-operative cases, all cases with ectopic glands, and in all patients with single-gland disease whereas in multi-gland disease, involvement of more than one gland was visualized in only 61% of the patients[21]. In a series of persistent or recurrent HPT cases, Numerow and co-authors also observed that MIBI accuracy was 94% for adenomas but 43% for hyperplasia [37]. In vitamin D deficiency, which causes parathyroid hyperplasia, there is a greater tracer uptake with improved sensitivity of Sestamibi in patients with primary HPT that are vitamin D deficient[38]. In univariate analysis, the mean weight of secondary hyperplastic glands detected by MIBI prior to initial surgery was higher than for undetected glands[36] and visualized adenomas are heavier than those not depicted by MIBI in cases re-operated for persistent HPT[26]. There is a similar association between adenoma weight and positive MIBI scans in previously unoperated primary HPT patients[33,34] and it has also been shown that parathyroid volume is inversely related to vitamin D levels[39]. In accordance with other series,[7,26,28,33,34] ectopic location and preoperative calcium or PTH were also not associated with MIBI failure. It has been suggested that thyroid nodules may affect MIBI failure with thyroid adenomas causing false positive results [31,40].

Ectopic location was associated with failure of combined US and MIBI, with patients having ectopic glands presenting 15.5 higher odds for non-successful localization by both modalities than patients with orthotopic glands.[28]. Our result could, at least in part, be explained by the fact that half of combined US and MIBI failures indicated ectopic hyperplastic parathyroid glands. A high index of suspicion for ectopic location is therefore suggested in patients with both negative US and MIBI studies. This suspicion should be even higher in patients with persistent primary or secondary HPT, as shown by the multivariate analysis for predictors of ectopic location.

Selective Venous Sampling and Parathyroid Angiography

This technique is very difficult to accomplish and time consuming to perform. It involves cannulating multiple small veins. Localisation is assisted by angiography and the two should be considered as one investigation (figures 11.4 and 11.5).

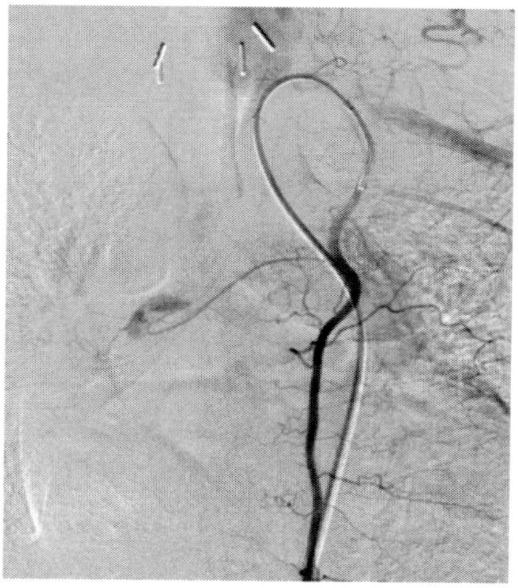

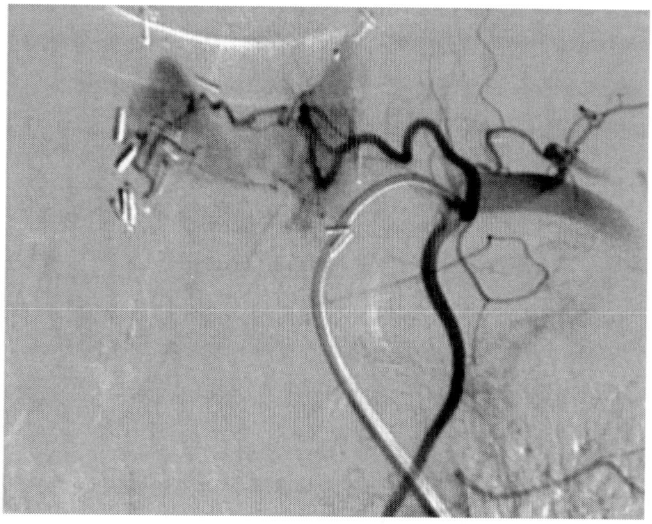

Figure 11. 4. shows the result of parathyroid angiography with the vascular blush clearly visible. Figure 11.5. shows the detailed vein mapping required.

However, angiography does have a very small risk of embolisation and arterial thrombosis which in the neck can lead to CVA. Its use therefore needs considered justification. No predictors of selective venous sampling and parathyroid angiography failure were found in this study while the very few unsuccessful results of combined selective venous sampling and parathyroid angiography prohibited further analysis for identification of risk factors of both modalities failure. Whether previous thyroid surgery confounds selective venous sampling is unproven as the 2 studies that have looked at this had conflicting results[11,15]. Previous neck operations with vessel ligation distort the cervical vascular anatomy making them more challenging to catheterize and may result in a more difficult interpretation of selective venous sampling and parathyroid angiography results. Previous thyroid or parathyroid surgery does not significantly affect the high success rate of these methods as when they are combined the sensitivity is 91-95%[41], when the investigation is performed by interventional radiologists with high levels of expertise and experience. Careful mapping is needed to enable correlation of PTH sample results and anatomy using veins cannulated during the procedure and the localisation found on angiography (figures 11.6 and 11.7).

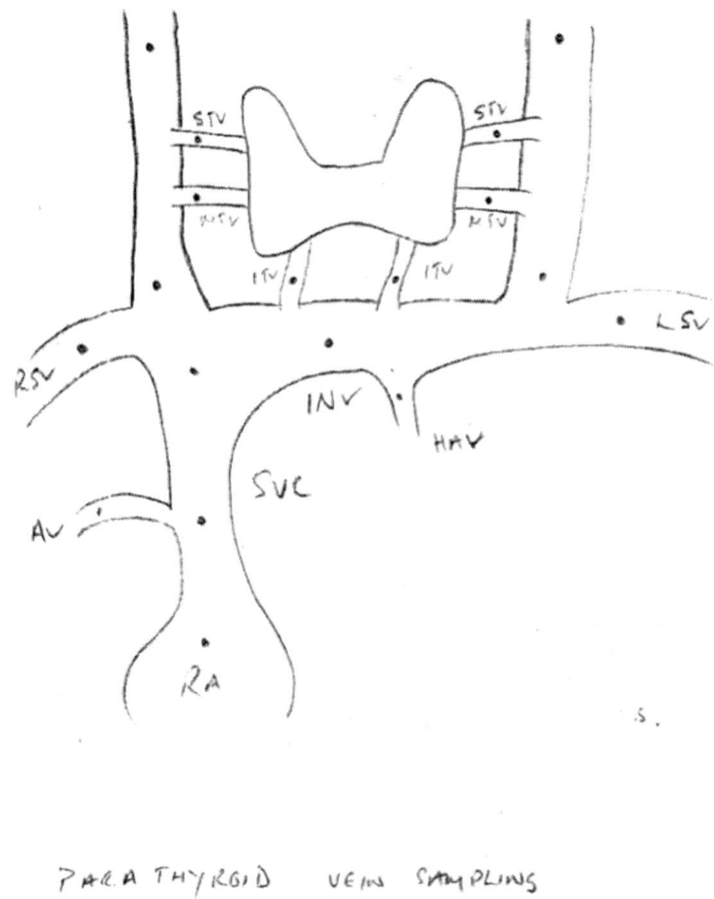

Figure 11.6. (Continued next page)

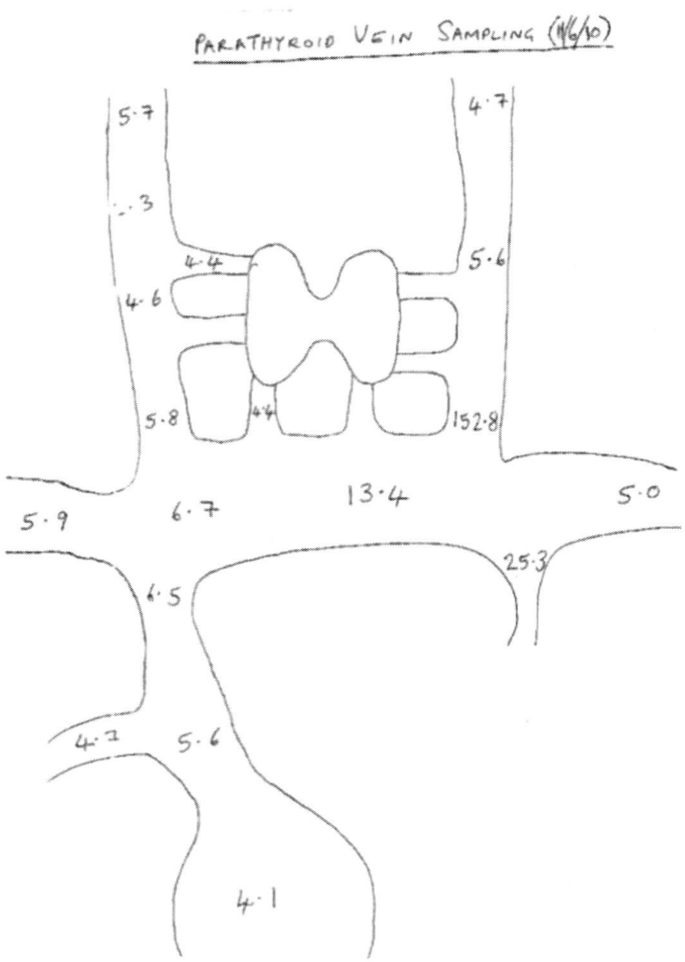

Figure 11.6. and 11.7. shows an example of vein mapping with PTH sample results that reveal the location of the parathyroid adenoma.

Conclusion

Despite the high success rates at the initial operation by experienced surgeons, some persistent or recurrent cases of hyperparathyroidism are inevitable. Meticulous preoperative investigation is crucial for providing maximum information prior to re-operation, thus allowing for an effective surgical approach and successful treatment of these patients. Appropriate interpretation of preoperative imaging studies and knowledge of the potential location of abnormal parathyroid glands can lead to very high cure rates with minimal morbidity. The identified predictors of ectopic gland location and failure of imaging methods in patients with persistent or recurrent HPT are particularly useful for interpreting imaging results and planning operative strategy in this challenging group of patients. Combined venous sampling and parathyroid angiography is probably the most helpful procedure to aid localisation when available.

References

[1] Hedbäck G, Odén A. Persistent disease after surgery for primary hyperparathyroidism: the long-term outcome. *Eur. J. Endocrinol.* 2004; 150:19-25.

[2] Hedbäck G, Odén A. Recurrence of hyperparathyroidism; a long-term follow-up after surgery for primary hyperparathyroidism. *Eur. J. Endocrinol.* 2003; 148:413-421.

[3] Caron NR, Sturgeon C, Clark OH. Persistent and recurrent hyperparathyroidism. *Curr. Treat Options Oncol.* 2004; 5:335-345.

[4] Wells SA Jr, Debenedetti MK, Doherty GM. Recurrent or persistent hyperparathyroidism. *J. Bone Miner. Res.* 2002; 17 Suppl 2:N158-162.

[5] Weber CJ, Sewell CW, McGarity WC. Persistent and recurrent sporadic primary hyperparathyroidism: histopathology, complications, and results of re-operation. *Surgery* 1994; 116:991-998.

[6] Arnalsteen L, Quievreux JL, Huglo D, Pattou F, Carnaille B, Proye C. Reoperation for persistent or recurrent primary hyperparathyroidism. Seventy-seven cases among 1888 operated patients. *Ann. Chir.* 2004; 129:224-231.

[7] Hibi Y, Tominaga Y, Sato T, Katayama A, Haba T, Uchida K, Ichimori T, Numano M, Tanaka Y, Takagi H, Imai T, Funahashi H, Nakao A. Re-operation for renal hyperparathyroidism. *World J. Surg.* 2002; 26:1301-1307.

[8] Mariette C, Pellissier L, Combemale F, Quievreux JL, Carnaille B, Proye C. Re-operation for persistent or recurrent primary hyperparathyroidism. *Langenbecks Arch. Surg.* 1998; 383:174-179.

[9] McGarity WC, Goldman AL. Re-operation for primary hyperparathyroidism. *Ann. Surg.* 1981; 194:134-139.

[10] Udelsman R, Donovan PI. Remedial parathyroid surgery: changing trends in 130 consecutive cases. *Ann. Surg.* 2006; 244:471-479.

[11] Reidel MA, Schilling T, Graf S, Hinz U, Nawroth P, Büchler MW, Weber T. Localization of hyper-functioning parathyroid glands by selective venous sampling in reoperation for primary or secondary hyperparathyroidism. *Surgery* 2006; 140:907-913; discussion 913.

[12] Billings PJ, Milroy EJ. Re-operative parathyroid surgery. *Br. J. Surg.* 1983; 70:542-546.

[13] Gough I. Re-operative parathyroid surgery: the importance of ectopic location and multi-gland disease. *ANZ J. Surg.* 2006; 76:1048-1050.

[14] Silver CE, Velez FJ. Parathyroid re-exploration. *Am. J. Surg.* 1992; 164:606-609.

[15] Jones JJ, Brunaud L, Dowd CF, Duh QY, Morita E, Clark OH. Accuracy of selective venous sampling for intact parathyroid hormone in difficult patients with recurrent or persistent hyperparathyroidism. *Surgery* 2002; 132:944-950; discussion 950-951.

[16] Estella E, Leong MS, Bennett I, Hartley L, Wetzig N, Archibald CA, Harper JS, Cuneo RC. Parathyroid hormone venous sampling prior to reoperation for primary hyperparathyroidism. *ANZ J. Surg.* 2003; 73:800-805.

[17] Seehofer D, Steinmüller T, Rayes N, Podrabsky P, Riethmüller J, Klupp J, Ulrich F, Schindler R, Frei U, Neuhaus P. Parathyroid hormone venous sampling before re-operative surgery in renal hyperparathyroidism: comparison with noninvasive localization procedures and review of the literature. *Arch. Surg.* 2004; 139:1331-1338.

[18] Shen W, Düren M, Morita E, Higgins C, Duh QY, Siperstein AE, Clark OH. Reoperation for persistent or recurrent primary hyperparathyroidism. *Arch. Surg.* 1996; 131:861-867; discussion 867-869.

[19] Jaskowiak N, Norton JA, Alexander HR, Doppman JL, Shawker T, Skarulis M, Marx S, Spiegel A, Fraker DL. A prospective trial evaluating a standard approach to re-operation for missed parathyroid adenoma. *Ann. Surg.* 1996; 224:308-320; discussion 320-321.

[20] Hessman O, Stålberg P, Sundin A, Garske U, Rudberg C, Eriksson LG, Hellman P, Akerström G. High success rate of parathyroid re-operation may be achieved with improved localization diagnosis. *World J. Surg.* 2008; 32:774-781; discussion 782-783.

[21] Caixàs A, Bernà L, Hernández A, Tébar FJ, Madariaga P, Vegazo O, Bittini AL, Moreno B, Faure E, Abós D, Piera J, Rodríguez JM, Farrerons J, Puig-Domingo M. Efficacy of preoperative diagnostic imaging localization of technetium 99m-sestamibi scintigraphy in hyperparathyroidism. *Surgery* 1997; 121:535-541.

[22] Wang CA. Parathyroid re-exploration. A clinical and pathological study of 112 cases. *Ann. Surg.* 1977; 186:140-145.

[23] Thompson GB, Grant CS, Perrier ND, Harman R, Hodgson SF, Ilstrup D, van Heerden JA. Re-operative parathyroid surgery in the era of sestamibi scanning and intra-operative parathyroid hormone monitoring. *Arch. Surg.* 1999; 134:699-704; discussion 704-705.

[24] Roslyn JJ, Mulder DG, Gordon HE. Persistent and recurrent hyperparathyroidism. *Am. J. Surg.* 1981; 142:21-25.

[25] Hasse C, Sitter H, Brune M, Wollenteit I, Nies C, Rothmund M. Quality of life and patient satisfaction after re-operation for primary hyperparathyroidism: analysis of long-term results. *World J. Surg.* 2002; 26:1029-1036.

[26] Nilsson B, Fjälling M, Klingenstierna H, Mölne J, Jansson S, Tisell LE. Effects of preoperative parathyroid localisation studies on the cost of operations for persistent hyperparathyroidism. *Eur. J. Surg.* 2001; 167: 587-591.

[27] Rodriguez JM, Tezelman S, Siperstein AE, Duh QY, Higgins C, Morita E, Dowd CF, Clark OH. Localization procedures in patients with persistent or recurrent hyperparathyroidism. *Arch. Surg.* 1994; 129:870-875.

[28] Feingold DL, Alexander HR, Chen CC, Libutti SK, Shawker TH, Simonds WF, Marx SJ, Skarulis MC, Doppman JL, Schrump DS, Bartlett DL. Ultrasound and sestamibi scan as the only preoperative imaging tests in reoperation for parathyroid adenomas. *Surgery* 2000; 128:1103-1109; discussion 1109-1110.

[29] Reading CC, Charboneau JW, James EM, Karsell PR, Grant CS, van Heerden JA, Purnell DC. Postoperative parathyroid high-frequency sonography: evaluation of persistent or recurrent hyperparathyroidism. *AJR Am. J. Roentgenol* 1985; 144:399-402.

[30] Lake E, Kirkby-Bott J, Jackson J Palazzo F. Manubrial split provides adequate exposure for mediastinal exploration for parathyroid adenoma. *Endocrine abstracts* 2008; 18:26.

[31] Prinz RA, Lonchina V, Carnaille B, Wurtz A, Proye C. Thorascopic excision of enlarged mediastinal parathyroid glands. *Surgery* 1994; 116:999-1005.

[32] Ghaheri BA, Koslin DB, Wood AH, Cohen JI. Preoperative ultrasound is worthwhile for re-operative parathyroid surgery. *Laryngoscope* 2004; 114:2168-2171.

[33] Erbil Y, Barbaros U, Yanik BT, Salmaslioğlu A, Tunaci M, Adalet I, Bozbora A, Ozarmağan S. Impact of gland morphology and concomitant thyroid nodules on preoperative localization of parathyroid adenomas. *Laryngoscope* 2006; 116:580-585.

[34] Erbil Y, Barbaros U, Tükenmez M, Işsever H, Salmaslioğlu A, Adalet I, Ozarmağan S, Tezelman S . Impact of adenoma weight and ectopic location of parathyroid adenoma on localization study results. *World J. Surg.* 2008; 32:566-571.

[35] O'Doherty MJ, Kettle AG, Wells P, Collins RE, Coakley AJ. Parathyroid imaging with technetium-99m-sestamibi: preoperative localization and tissue uptake studies. *J. Nucl. Med.* 1992; 33:313-318.

[36] Pham TH, Sterioff S, Mullan BP, Wiseman GA, Sebo TJ, Grant CS. Sensitivity and utility of parathyroid scintigraphy in patients with primary versus secondary and tertiary hyperparathyroidism. *World J. Surg.* 2006; 30:327-332.

[37] Numerow LM, Morita ET, Clark OH, Higgins CB. Persistent/recurrent hyperparathyroidism: a comparison of sestamibi scintigraphy, MRI, and ultrasonography. *J. Magn. Reson Imaging.* 1995; 5:702-708.

[38] Kandil E, Tufaro AP, Carson KA, Lin F, Somervell H, Farrag T Dackiw A, Zeiger M, Tufano RP. Correlation of plasma 25-Hydroxyvitamin D levels with severity of primary HPT and likelihood of parathyroid adenoma localization on sestamibi scan. *Arch. Otolaryngol. Head Neck Surg.* 2008;134(10):1071-5.

[39] J.Kirkby-Bott, Z El-Khatib, B Soudan, R Caiazzo, L Arnalsteen, B Carnaille. *25 hydroxy vitamin D deficiency causes parathyroid incidentalomas. Langenbeck Arch. Surg,*(2010). 395; 919-924. DOI: 10.1007/s00423-010-0692-4.

[40] Inabnet WB, Lee JA, Henry JF, Sebag F. Parathyroid Disease; Part 1. In Lennard TWJ, editor. *A companion to specialist surgical practice: Endocrine Surgery.* Edinburgh: Saunders Elsevier; 2009;1-38.

[41] Miller DL. Preoperative localisation and interventional treatment of parathyroid tumours: when and how? *World J. Surg.* 1991;15:706.

Index

C

D

E

F

G

H

I

J

K

L

M

N

O

P

Q

R

S

T

U

V

W

Y